The CHRONICLES of PAIN

JASON GOODMAN

Life swings like a pendulum backward
And forward between pain and boredom.

— Arthur Schopenhauer

The preponderance of pain over pleasure
is the cause of our fictitious morality
and religion.

— Friedrich Nietzsche

Additional books by Jason Goodman:

Blood on My Hands and a Knife in My Back

Simple Reflections on a Frozen Surface

Nervous Reader

Nervous Reader/Second Edition

a. PUZZLED EXISTENCE

Urban Gothic

Urban Gothic 2

Copyright 2020 by Jason Goodman
First Printing 2021
Library of Congress PIN Number: 2021904641
ISBN Number: 978 0 578 84950 8

All rights reserved. No part of this book may be reproduced in either paper or digital format or used in any way. Nor may this material be downloaded into any form of information storage or retrieval system without the written permission of the author.

Available on Amazon.com
Kindle e-books
And wherever fine books are sold.

Front-cover design by: Alchemy Studio. Inc.
Back-cover photograph: Teresa Fee Goodman

DISCLAIMER:

The contents of this volume are based on my experiences as a patient who underwent a total of 45 major medical interventions. These consisted of surgeries, viral pneumonias, and issues related to my experience in combat during the Vietnam War. This also entailed the effects of exposure to Agent Orange and the Coronavirus. I am neither a doctor nor a pharmacist. I am an artist and writer and have been involved with those particular disciplines for more than 50 years. The stories and experiences that I have detailed in this book are based on my personal experience both in and recovering from prolonged hospitalizations.

This book represents a culmination of numerous acute observations over many days spent under professional hospital care.

Hopefully, my lifetime of experience and mistakes may help to pave a smoother transition for those who come after me and find themselves under the knife and confined to a bed.

INQUIRIES:

Alchemy Studio, Inc. Art & Design

Fine literary works

Lititz, Pennsylvania and Westport, Ireland

www.alchemystudioinc.com

Joshua Riggan
Graphic Design Studios

Frank W. Kresen
proof positive
Copy Editing/Proofreading
www.artisanproofpositive.com

Interior Layout Design:
Kimberly A. Walsh
Artisan Graphic Design
www.artisankimwalsh.com

Printed in the United States of America

Dedication

Dr. W. Clemens Rosenberger
April 18, 1932-January 27, 2021

The good doctor spoke of love, and I listened. We taught each other many things over the years, but I suspect that he gave more to the process than I. Clem was a good man, he enjoyed a good life, and now it has ended.

Missing this person is not the point. Being left partially filled with his wisdom is!

Reap your reward, my old friend, and be at peace.

Table of Contents:

Chapter One: Bent, Broken, and Busted
— Page 14
An apt description of methods that may warrant hospitalization and surgery.

Chapter Two: Drugs, Therapies, and Devices
— Page 54
An examination of various treatments for prolonged and chronic pain. The good, bad, and downright ugly in the realm of opioid medications.

Chapter Three: Backless Gowns, Bad Beds, and Jello
— Page 84
The hospitalization experience from inside, along with the importance of leaving your dignity at the hospital's front door.

Chapter Four: Days and Nights with the Coronavirus
— Page 130
A personal reflection on the effects of infection with a virus of deadly consequences, from two completely different perspectives.

Chapter Five: The Dreaded Follow-Up Visit
— Page 168
What happens after you leave the hospital and how it impacts your life for many weeks and months afterward.

Chapter Six: Give Us Today Our Daily *Pain*
— 182
An examination of various ways to live with extreme, chronic pain and realizing that there just may be alternative methods for dealing with it.

Chapter One

Bent, Broken, and Busted

The Chronicles of Pain

I actually don't have any recall about my first encounter with pain. I was around two years old when this hideous accident occurred. The story that my mother explained to me went like this.

She had me outside, in a crib of sorts, to enjoy the summer air. Somehow, I managed to escape the confines of my prison and decided to explore my surroundings. I was supposedly crawling up my dad's dirt driveway when it happened. Back in those days, we were a very poor family. My father worked as a coal miner in one of the many mines that the Wilkes-Barre area had to offer. My family lived on the side of an undeveloped mountain, and there was a dirt road leading up to the house. In fact, now that I think of it, everything was dirt around our house, including the driveway. As the years ticked by, our fortunes changed, and all of that dirt would be surfaced with macadam once we became very wealthy. But, in 1952, there was a lot of dirt.

Being that we lived on the side of a mountain, the topology had a distinct slant to it, mainly downward. So, the driveway was full of ruts that were created when the rains came and made their own path to the bottom of this mountain road. I was told that I crawled into one of these ruts in the road surface, and my father drove in and ran over me. Because I was in this rut, I wasn't squeezed like a pancake by the tire of his car. The walls of my rut stabilized and prevented the tire from reaching its bottom. Naturally, my mother screamed bloody murder, my father felt really bad (I think), and they rushed me to the doctor's office.

Back in those days, you weren't taken to a doctor unless internal organs were gushing out of your various orifices. The old sawbones supposedly rolled me around and poked at my body, using his highly trained fingers to deduce that nothing of importance was severely damaged. This, of course, relieved my dad's guilt and allowed him to shout at my mother the entire trip home about her skill as such. What was not discovered during the examination was the condition of the various vertebrae located in my lower back. Some of them had been compromised by my ordeal.

The problem with the lumbar region is that damage can sometimes be insidious. An example of this would be a hip pain being mimicked as lower back pain, and vice-versa. Damage to this part of the back, in the L4, L5, S1, S2 region, will be amplified by certain movements — shoveling, sweeping, raking, any activity that required a twist. Damn that Chubby Checker and his music.

The pain was always there; the only thing

The Chronicles of Pain

that changed was its intensity. During those early years, a complaint of that nature was always dismissed as an excuse to avoid work, and work was the most important thing in my father's universe.

Early on, when I served with the U.S. Navy, they stationed me at the now-defunct Philadelphia Naval Shipyard. In the barracks, they always posted a watch. I don't mean the device you wear on your wrist — it was a person assigned to keep an eye on things. You never knew when a KGB agent would show up and try to steal the pillows and blankets from our bunks. A watch usually lasted for four hours, and they could be at any time of the day or night. When I was given the "dead man's" watch, which is 12:00 midnight to 4:00 a.m., my back would scream at me. Besides being a "dead man's" watch, it was also a "roving" watch. This meant I had to constantly walk around and punch various timing and verification devices, which served as proof of where I was, or, basically, if I was doing my job. Walking four solid hours on those tile floors was killing me.

So, one day I went to the corpsman, the Navy's version of a medical clinic, and spoke to a doctor. I went through my entire story of woe, embellished, of course, with having to wrestle KGB agents to the floor on a regular basis, but he didn't believe me.

Which is another important point of being a person who suffers from chronic back pain. Practically no one ever believes you when you tell them how bad your back hurts, especially if there is a workman's compensation attorney involved.

Anyway, back to the Navy. My "rating," which is your job classification in the Navy, was that of a "Boatswain's Mate." We were the guys who chipped and painted the ship. We were also assigned to guns occasionally and making sure that the boat didn't sink, also known as "Damage Control." I began to have doubts about being in this position because it entailed a lot of work, but, more importantly, it always involved standing watch. I was not interested in leaving the Navy — that was the last thing on my mind. But this doctor thought I was trying to dodge the draft, even though I had enlisted in the service of my own accord. It was 1969, and they needed anyone with a pulse to throw at the little scrimmage in Vietnam. This guy had that look of complete disdain on his face. You could see the word "coward" in the thought balloon above his head.

I simply wanted to explore the possibility of changing my rating, or "job," if you prefer. I asked if I could take the "Journalism" course that the Navy offered and become a star reporter for the "*Don't Pick up the Soap News.*"[1] This position would have placed me behind a desk somewhere banging out Pulitzer-prize-winning stories and articles. As fate would have it, the doctor was a Marine. That may not sound like much to you, but when you are in the Navy and you encounter someone in the Marines, you immediately must get into a vicious fistfight. The Marines have this undying hatred for anyone or anything associated with the U.S. Navy. If you really want to piss off a Marine, just tell him to look at his paycheck, especially the part that says, "Department of the Navy"!

This guy just assumed that I was gay and wanted to go home to mother. That was the reality of those days. I don't know if it has changed or not, but a Marine is always a Marine; even if he's dead, trust me — he would still hate the Navy guys.

My entire effort that day warranted orders to Vietnam. At the time, all of my MMPI test results told everyone I had a problem with authority figures. Consequently, this Marine quack and I went round and round in a somewhat heated display of anger. He outranked me, and, so, it turned out to be an exercise in futility. This, of course, doomed me to years of pain.

I experienced constant low-volume pain at that time. The pain was there when I awoke, and the pain just got louder and louder as the

---
[1] This is an insider reference to a small, sick, Navy joke.

day progressed. This led to a titanic struggle just to fall asleep that evening. It went on day after day — *24/7*, as our current Newspeak would express it.

My situation got much worse after a fall onto a metal deck. We were motoring up the Mekong River one day and came under mortar attack. In order to avoid a direct hit, the officers proceeded to engage in a zig-zag maneuver, a practice that is usually reserved for evading submarines — out on the open ocean. This maneuver was not designed to be used in a shallow river. We ran aground, abruptly, and I was thrown off a ladder, where I'd been engaged in damage control below the water line. I fell backwards about eight feet and landed on my back. After this incident, I pretty much needed pain medication on a daily basis just to take the sharp edges off the signals going to my brain. It more or less removed all of the politically incorrect curse words from my spinal column.

It is an interesting testimony to the Vietnam War: Everyone there was high on something most of the time. You *had* to be stoned to maintain even a modicum of reality. For me, it was the Darvon "Pearls" and a can of beer that permeated my daily routine. Back in those days, Darvon, the least-effective painkiller on anyone's scale, had a small, black sphere inside — the "pearl" — surrounded by white powder

The Chronicles of Pain

that was basically a placebo, or just aspirin. You would pull the capsule apart and extract the little black ball, dilute it in a can of beer, and then experience a few hours without nerve-shattering pain. It was some pretty low-grade stuff and the only thing the Navy dispensed at the time. Darvon has now fallen out of favor and has been replaced by another product, called "Darvocet." It is the same compound, only the black pearl has been incorporated into the mixture. These are the bottom of the pain-medication food chain. If you suffer from chronic pain, the Darvon family of drugs quickly outlive their effectiveness.

After returning from the Vietnam War, I lived on a diet of Tylenol 3 and 4 when they were available. Back in the early 1970s, there weren't too many physicians dispensing opiate-based medications. So, when you *did* manage to procure a prescription, it wouldn't have many refills on the label. I had to stretch out every pill, usually saving them for later in the evening.

Another incident that occurred that exacerbated my pain levels involved an accident with a motorcycle and an automobile. Guess who lost?

I was discharged from the Navy on July 20, 1970, at Treasure Island in San Francisco. The Navy maintained a small base there, right below one of those giant pylons that hold up the Oakland Bay Bridge. My discharge was a case of *Here's your hat — don't let the door hit you in the ass on your way out.* I wasn't alone. A number of the military services did this to their personnel after the Vietnam War. You almost got the impression that you had been used and then discarded. It happened to a number of people I knew in the various Vietnam Veteran organizations that I belonged to back in those days. They knew what they were doing. I think they realized the VA healthcare system was going to be swamped with returning service members needing to be repaired both physically and mentally. (We won't go into the emotional side of it!)

I remember the procedure well: An officer would ask if you wanted to be discharged from the Navy. Now, think about that: You just returned from the hell of jungle warfare, and there always was a remote possibility that they would send you back, so the answer to that question, you would think, was quite obvious. Then, just to round things out, they would sneak little provisions into your discharge papers. Usually these dealt with the prospects of receiving VA benefits. I know this because it actually happened to me. I was listed as a "medical release" and *not entitled* to any benefits; naturally, this information came much

The Chronicles of Pain

later. So, I accepted their offer and received a plane ticket and $91 for my trouble.

It was September 1970 when I made it back to Pennsylvania. I purchased a 500cc Triumph motorcycle. It was sweet. I bought it from a newbie lawyer whose wife was pregnant; he needed the money. That is something else I have seen often: As soon as little Johnny comes along, the husband has to sell his motorcycle. I guess the fear of losing a breadwinner outweighs the man's desire to own a nice machine. Anyway, it might be best to leave that line of reasoning alone before I type myself into a MADD contingent on my doorstep!

So, I bought the thing, and it turned out to be one of the best investments I ever made. That bike never let me down. I decided to forgo owning a car and rode that machine everywhere and in every kind of weather. For an entire year of rain, snow, dust storms, and wild beasts chasing me, I simply rode on. There was a reason for this madness.

I sailed LST 902 back from Vietnam; it was an old leftover from WW2. The trip required 58 days at sea to accomplish this feat. Those old rust-bucket LSTs (Landing Ship Tank) had a flat bottom, so they could operate in any kind of shallow water, as in the Mekong River. The boats were built very cheaply because they weren't expected to last very long off Okinawa.

A good number of them succumbed to artillery fire, *kamikaze* attacks, and foul seas. We sailed that tub across the Pacific Ocean right into Vallejo, California, where it was to be scrapped and turned into Toyota parts or razor blades. Usually, when your ship is scrapped out from underneath you, they will give you a choice as to where you will serve next. I picked a small submarine base on the coast of Scotland, and I saved up all of my leave, all 30 days of it. My plan was to buy a brand-new BSA or Triumph motorcycle and ride it around Europe for a month. Maybe now, you can understand my rationale for buying a motorcycle at the time.

Well, I rode that bike a lot, running out to Long Island to visit my girlfriend at the time, Meredith. She lived in Setauket, out there by Stony Brook. Let me tell you — it was a very cold ride in November from Wilkes-Barre, Pennsylvania, to the end of Long Island.

The better part of a year passed, and my thoughts changed about owning a motorcycle over a car. I decided to sell the bike and buy a nice little Mustang or something similar. I sold the bike to my good friend Carl, and he was coming to pick it up the next day. Man, that thing looked good! I had shined it up and cleaned every little detail; it sat there in the doorway of my art studio just begging me to take it out for "one more ride." Please, don't ever fall for that "one more ride" trick — it can prove to be fatal.

In that accident, I wasn't killed, but I was damaged fairly well. There wasn't anyone else on the road besides me and a huge Oldsmobile "88." Younger people won't know what an Oldsmobile 88 was, but I can describe it like this: Picture an aircraft carrier with four wheels, and then put a chrome sign on it that says, "88."

The wreck put me in the hospital for a few days with various structural injuries, mainly my knees and shoulders. Picture a man flying over a car while seated on a motorcycle and you will see the position my body was in when I hit the pavement. It turned out to be just a little more pain for me to deal with, on top of the lower-back pain and just the act of getting up in the morning.

The Veterans Administration medical facilities use a pain-assessment system on a 1-to-10 scale, and then they throw in these tiny smiley faces that go from a smile to a deep frown. Well, that little "accident" sent my number from a solid 4 up into the 6s and 7s.

In the early '80s, my wife, Teresa, and I moved to Key West, Florida. I had lived in South Florida on and off for about 16 years. Most of my university work was done at Florida Atlantic University in Boca Raton — a town whose name translates into "the mouth of the rat…" During those mid-to-late '80s years, I lived and worked in that area. One of the jobs that I always fell back on was my ability to operate heavy equipment — bulldozers, backhoes, and that sort of thing. I actually helped to ruin a number of places by building ground where cheap homes would be placed, allowing a number of people from Ohio, New Jersey, and other locales in the North to live out their "golden" years in a warmer climate. The trouble with working in Florida was the fact that Florida is a "Right to Work" state. What that means is that the Florida sunshine is factored into your paycheck to the tune of 50 percent.

For example, in the mid-1970s, I was making union scale while working in Colorado — $15.84 per hour with benefits. Then, in Florida, in the late '70s and early '80s, I was being paid a maximum of $7.25 per hour and reminded that I was lucky to have a job. They would always say that they could get "some Haitian" to do the job for $4 an hour. And that is exactly what happened in Key West. My first job paid $6.25 an hour to start. It is something that I never understood — they give you a half-million-dollar machine, expect you not to damage the thing, and then pay you a paltry six bucks an hour. It never made any sense to me

The Chronicles of Pain

in all of the years I worked down there.

I had to work in Florida. My father refused to pay for college unless I stayed in Wilkes-Barre, Pennsylvania. That was not going to happen — once I found out that there were places where it didn't snow, I wasn't going to live in Wilkes-Barre, Pennsylvania. It was as simple as that! On top of that, the VA decided to contest my college benefits, which was the only reason I enlisted in the Navy, and, as it turned out, I was listed as "Black Ops" for the work we did in Vietnam. Black Ops means your entire military record is scrubbed of any incriminating evidence. An example of that would be going into Cambodia every month, when President Nixon was telling the American people we *weren't* in Cambodia. If the word got out, Washington would be embarrassed! My benefits, which I had earned under hostile gunfire, were cut or denied due to a president lying to his constituents.

There I was, years later, operating heavy equipment in Florida for a crummy $6.25 an hour, trying to earn enough money to return to college. I started working for one of the largest excavating companies in Key West. We were working on the expansion of Route 1 into the city. I was told to drive a water truck that had rolled over once before. The roof had been chopped off, and it lacked baffles in the

5,000 gallon water tank. This meant that, as I drove down the road, the truck would sway like a drunken sailor as the water sloshed around in the tank. One day, I backed up to a culvert to wet the shoulder when the damn thing rolled over again, throwing me out into the Mangrove swamp onto a pile of rocks. This accident injured — or should I say, re-injured — the same lower back area that had been affected in Vietnam, and the same place my father had conveniently crushed with his automobile. That accident turned up the pain level into the 9s.

It was May 26, 1986, when the company doctor, a golfing buddy of the owner, told me that nothing was wrong. I had simply "sprained" my back muscles. Naturally, I thought differently of his diagnosis, but, back then, you couldn't question the word of a "doctor." On one occasion, we almost came to blows when he accused me of "faking it" so that I could drink beer all day and not work. I tried to explain to him that my rent was $600 a month and that my workman's compensation came to $600 a month. I told him to do the math! Finally, I dared him to send me to Miami for an MRI. Three months later, after I'd suffered through Physical Therapy ("PT"), he relented.

That brings up a very good point. Why is it that, when you get injured, first, they don't

The Chronicles of Pain

believe you, and, next, they send you to PT? Keep in mind, I was really hurt. Pieces of my vertebrae were driven into my spinal column. The last thing I should have been doing was going to Physical Therapy and running the risk of being paralyzed! So, I drove myself to Miami, bad back and all, and had the MRI. The test results were sent to my "doctor" in Key West. This guy happened to be an orthopedic surgeon. Before I even got home, he'd called my wife and told her to bring me to the hospital the next morning because he had to perform "emergency surgery." Now, my wife is Irish; she didn't take the doctor's suggestion kindly and basically told him to stuff it. Little did he know, that, while I was in Miami, I had retained the services of a law firm that specialized in workman's compensation cases. This meant that there was a new sheriff in town.

A little word from experience: If you are injured on a job and know that you are hurt really bad, as soon as they start fucking with you, go out and get a good workman's compensation attorney. The doctor's attitude will change instantly, and the threats will stop immediately, because they know that a new voice is handling this accident. Another thing: Always get an accident report, and never — I repeat, *never* — lose the yellow and pink copy of that paperwork. It is possibly worth a lot of money, not to mention the medical care you will need for many years to come.

Under recommendation, I traveled to Scranton, Pennsylvania, and got a second opinion from a neurosurgeon. When it comes to a back injury, always consult a neurosurgeon — never an orthopedic guy. Don't hire a carpenter when you need an electrician!

Johnny Cash did a song years ago called "Ring of Fire," and one of the lines goes like this: *"Down, down, down/into a burning ring of fire/I fell into a burning ring of fire…"* It is the perfect analogy for chronic pain. The more surgeries you have to help relieve the pain, the more pain you get in return. My last neurosurgeon explained to me that we grow scar tissue on the inside of our body just like we do on the outside. After multiple back surgeries, the scar tissue displaces the nerves in the back, and that leads to complications, not to mention increased pain levels.

I ended up leaving Key West and flying up to Scranton, Pennsylvania. It was my "second opinion," after the debacle with the company orthopedic guy. I was introduced to Dr. Black, a neurosurgeon renowned for his work on the human brain. Dr. Black performed the first laminectomy in my lower back. I felt fairly good for a few months, but then my old nemesis returned with a vengeance. But, if I am to be perfectly honest with you, I did not follow the post-op regimen that the doctor had prescribed. I went out and did everything that a recent back-surgery patient should not do, and that undoubtedly led to my demise.

Now, that was my first lower-back surgery. I am going to jump ahead to my most recent one, in 2003. This doctor was something else. He was from India originally but had lived in the States for many years. He was like a Zen surgeon. His specialty was "invasive" surgery. Now that is the kind of person you need to talk to when considering the prospect of someone laying open your back. He was someone who would not do anything unless he was sure that he could fix something that is busted. Don't let anyone start sharpening their scalpel before you get a second opinion. Dr. Holla performed the last of six major surgeries on my back, and I remember a person telling me that *one* back surgery is *one too many*!

The day after Dr. Holla had operated on my back, I was lying in bed, and he popped in to see me. I said to him, "Hey, Doc. How did it go back there?" His commentary went like this: "Jason, it was like doing surgery at night, in a minefield, with a blindfold on. Nothing in your back is where it is supposed to be. What I estimated would take a maximum of one hour required more than four hours of steady work.

Please, don't let anyone cut on you again. I am surprised that you aren't in a wheelchair from all of the butcher work that they have done on you."

My next question was with regard to the pain. He told me that I would probably be on some form of pain medication for the rest of my life and that it would have to keep increasing in strength and dosage as time passed. As it turned out, my nerves were all entangled in and encased by the scar tissue. Because nothing was where it was supposed to be, I could expect really bad periods of leg spasms, neuropathy, and increased pain levels. Everything would vary in intensity and would never go away until the Big Sleep or a visit to The Neurosurgeon in the Sky. *"Down, down, down into a burning ring of fire..."*

Let me tell you about serious chronic pain; if you aren't interested, just flip a few pages. It is grossly misunderstood and usually under-medicated. Over the years, I have had three doctors apologize to me just before going into the operating room, because they thought that all of us chronic-pain people were on the take or trying to beat some insurance company out of their hard-earned money. (That was a joke!)

Usually, something actually *has* happened to people who suffer with chronic pain. One guy threw out his back on the golf course.

The Chronicles of Pain

The poor dear! Another one had a rotator-cuff injury; the pain literally drove him crazy. And the third, well, I'm not at liberty to say who. Let me just tell you this: He burned his copy of the *Kama Sutra* soon afterwards.

In 1988, I had just had surgery #2. My regular guy couldn't do it because he was a brain surgeon and had to fly to Ohio to save some young girl who got hurt in a car crash. This fill-in guy wasn't the master craftsman that the other guy was. He did a "by the book" laminectomy, but that turned out to be the problem. Allow me to explain. After this surgery, I returned to Boca Raton to complete two courses that were required for my teaching certificate. One day, I was walking from the parking lot to my class when I just fell over on my face. They rushed me to the hospital, and the doctor who worked on me is the whole point of this story.

The guy was a brilliant brain surgeon. He was also a multi-millionaire in his own right, mostly inherited money. He also owned a very expensive Italian sports car. He was reluctant to perform surgery on me because, in his own words, "I find these back surgeries to be rather boring…." That was until he found out that I knew a lot about cars. We sat there in that hospital room for about two hours talking about cars. After that, he agreed to do the surgery.

The next day, the sawbones came into my room and explained what had happened. I was told that the other guy had done, as I said before, a perfect, by-the-book laminectomy — but he didn't look to each side! When they take out disc material, eventually the vertebrae will drop down, because there is nothing to hold them up. That is what the donuts do. My vertebrae had dropped, and, on both sides, there were bone spurs that almost severed the nerves to my legs. The left leg was worse than the right. He told me that some of that nerve would come back, but not all of it, and that I would have trouble with my left leg for the rest of my life. After many months of Physical Therapy, I was taught to walk again.

I attempted to sue the guy who did the initial surgery. My endeavor had taken me to a big-shot Philadelphia lawyer's office. The attorney said, "If you find a neurosurgeon who will testify against another colleague, we will take the case...." I never did, and the statute of limitations ran out, leaving me with a constant pain problem to this very day.

Let me just say this: A critic might say, "What good would suing anyone do? You would still have the same amount of pain!" Well, it's a hell of a lot easier dealing with chronic pain when you have enough money to pay the rent. That is one insecurity that money can definitely help

The Chronicles of Pain

to correct. Granted, I'm not advocating just throwing out random lawsuits with the hope that one of them stick to a medical-malpractice insurance company. No. What I am saying is that, if you have been actually damaged by someone else's negligence, then you sue. The practical reason is this: That "damage" will be with you a long, long time.

One common technique to keep a vertebra from falling is called "fusion." Nope, it has nothing to do with modern jazz or the physics of thermonuclear events. It consists of placing a piece of bone, or coral, between the two vertebrae and allowing the body to knit that into a solid mass, connecting the two joints. When I had this done, they placed me in a brace, called a "Jewett brace." This thing was so uncomfortable to wear that they actually sent me to a 12-step-based self-help group for people in Jewett braces! It was absurd. The premise of this technique was to keep the spinal column from bending until this bone graft healed or was "welded" into the vertebrae.

The brace was like wearing a suit of armor. You could not take in a full breath when it was on, because it was that restrictive. I wore that fucking thing (that is the right adjective) for a total of 12 weeks! And I despised every minute of every day I had it on.

On the side of a Jewett brace is a provision

for installing a small padlock (I'm not making this up). My doctor said he could "trust" me to keep it on, but he did leave the lock off so that I could take a shower without the brace. Don't quote me on this, because, maybe, medical technology has come a long way since then, but this was the way a fusion surgery was dealt with in the healing stages. The Jewett brace would be right at home in Nuremburg, that Bavarian town where medieval torture was performed.

I mentioned "coral" earlier, in the same sentence that the word "fusion" appeared. They were experimenting with a certain type of coral as a substitute for real bone — either your own bone, extracted from another part of your body, or cadaver bone. The bone from your own body works best because the body doesn't reject it as quickly, but the drawback there is the size of the piece required. It wouldn't make much sense to cut off a leg just to get enough bone to patch up your back!

From 2004 until 2010, I was given a respite from back surgery — but only because other parts of my body started to fail. I developed numb areas in my arms, and it got progressively worse; soon the numbness had overtaken my hands and fingers. The problems came to light while I was painting in Ireland; the brushes started to fly out of my hands. At first, I thought there was something on my fingers, but repeated

The Chronicles of Pain

washing of my hands never solved the problem. After we returned from Ireland and Mexico, where we go in the winter, and after the death of both my father and older brother, I began the process with the Veterans Administration to take a look at this issue.

Meanwhile, I started to experience electric shocks in my right arm. They would begin in my shoulder and shoot down my arm, into my hand, and right out of my fingertips. Again, it started out very mildly and gradually grew more violent and extremely painful. After a few years of MRIs and EMGs and one ulnar surgery, I was finally sent to the Hershey Medical Center in Hershey, Pennsylvania, to have surgery on my neck in the "C" sections. I don't mean to sound ungrateful, but it turned into another medical nightmare of Gothic proportions, similar to many others I've had to date. My doctor was a young lion who never spoke directly to Teresa or myself; he went through an assistant who stood a few feet away from him. It was stupid — like something out of the movies. He would tell the PA, and then that guy would tell us the same thing. We were sitting a few feet away as this exchange went on — it was really weird stuff! (I elaborate on this incident in Chapter Five.)

If there is one absolute truth that I would stake my life on, it is this: Doctors, especially neurosurgeons, are not infallible. Naturally, if asked, they would beg to differ, but if a mistake is made, they would deny any responsibility — it is *never* their fault. The problem with this line of reasoning is that I am a living example of its falsity.

A total of three interventions were done on my neck. While that surgery was happening, another team was doing another ulnar-nerve adjustment. It was like Henry Ford's $5-a-day assembly line. Just think: Four neurosurgeries being accomplished at one time — incredible! After I awoke, my right arm did not function at all. It required 10 days of phone calls to find out why this was. I honestly wish this was a piece of fiction, but it isn't. Three months of PT three times a week, and I couldn't touch the top of my head with my right arm. I worked out with an eight-pound dumbbell for the next nine months to achieve full range of motion. After each workout, the pain showed up, like clockwork. I'd sit around wondering when it was going to show up: *The pain — there has to be pain.*

"Down, down, down/into that burning ring of fire...." Chronic, severe pain of this type is conducive to thinking about taking oneself out. It isn't uncommon to think that way; I've done it on several occasions. Fortunately, I never actually put that plan in motion. Just idly

The Chronicles of Pain

mentioning the big "S" word in the wrong place will guarantee a 72-hour trip to the booby hatch. So, be careful what you say in mixed company — or around a wife or husband who is trying to do away with you for insurance reasons. I have been there and never done it. One big consideration was the mess that someone would have to clean up if I popped a .38 into my head. Another issue was the prospect of my wife not receiving my life insurance. I know what death looks like, especially a violent one, and it's not very nice, I won't even use the term "not pretty" because that doesn't even scratch the surface of its depravity. It is something that never goes away, even at three in the morning. No pill or any amount of liquor will ever make that vision go away.

Please bear with me as I relate a little story concerning the topic of suicide. My wife and I lived in Charleston, South Carolina, from 1990 to 1996. We had an old beach house on Folly Island. From my studio windows, I could look out over the Atlantic Ocean.

Basically, you could say that I was either very lucky or that I may have been in the right place at the right time. I started an advertising agency, and, after a few months, I could not believe how successful this little business was becoming. After about a year, I had about eight clients and a few heavy hitters that spent a lot of money on their advertising budgets. My wife took care of the paperwork, and I did the rest of the work.

One of my clients was located in Greenville, South Carolina. I would drive up there and spend a few nights in a hotel. My dealings were with the local Fox affiliate, Fox 21. I started to make television commercials and found out that I was pretty good at it. Naturally, my client insisted on starring in his own commercials, — as Andy Warhol would say, "their 15 minutes of fame." Actually, the ads were usually 15- and 30-second spots. I also did radio and print ads. For the television work, I ended up purchasing ad schedules, which entailed spending a huge sum of my man's money. But they paid off! His business started to flourish, and so did mine. Everything I did was billable, from the storyboards for the TV ads, to the print ad fonts. At one point, I hired a sound studio and a musician to make my own "music beds." When you build a television ad, you can't throw just anybody's music in the background, due to copyright laws. Most of the "canned" music was pretty weak, so I decided to make my own background music. Any ads that Alchemy Studio did had a distinct sound to them.

Things were going really well; we were making a lot of money, and my investments prospered. The only fly in the ointment, as old folks would say, were the leg problems. Practically every night, I would awaken at all hours with these horrendous leg spasms. They felt like someone was turning a hot screw down the middle of my leg bones; the pain was absolutely incredible. I would have to jump out of bed and stand against the wall to push my feet down onto the floor and try to prevent some of the pain. One night I actually timed the length of one of my leg spasms; it turned out that it lasted 18 minutes — 18 minutes of sheer agony. What became a really insidious problem was making love to my wife. Right at the critical moment, both of my legs would cramp up, and I had to jump out of bed with my johnson bobbing around and bouncing off the wall. Actually, it wasn't very funny at the time, but now that I look back on it, I *have* to make light of the situation.

So, the advertising agency continued to make a ton of money, and the spasms, well, they continued, too. I was also involved in a workman's compensation settlement dating back to the accident in Key West and my hotshot Miami lawyer. We were discussing the possibility of settling the medical portion of my claim, but before that happened, Teresa convinced me to go get a second opinion from the supposedly best place in the country, The Mayo Clinic. So, I flew out to Minnesota and booked a hotel room in Rochester. That is how you do it. If you are walking wounded, they ask you to stay in a hotel across the street; then you attend your appointments from there. At my first appointment, I explained as best I could to the doctor my situation with these cramps. I also mentioned the problems with my love making because it happened just about every single time. This doctor laughed and then said, "Well, that's easy to fix — I'll just write a prescription banning any form of sex...."

Ha, ha, ha.

I went *nuts*. When a combat veteran of Vietnam goes nuts, it's not a pretty sight. I started to curse like a sailor, which is what I was for a few years, and stormed out of this clown's office. You see, I'd heard that "joke" before, and it was wearing thin on my nerves. I didn't fly halfway across the country to hear it again — especially from the *esteemed* Mayo Clinic.

But this is to be expected. I hate to say this, but, if you are new to the chronic-pain life, you have to get used to ass-hat doctors who say really stupid things. It goes with the territory.

So, they did a whole bunch of tests, using me as a demonstration-model pin cushion for their EEGs. I'm dead serious. I was being administered EEGs and noticed that the faces kept changing. Have you ever had an EEG?

The Chronicles of Pain

They are terrible. They stick a needle into your ankle or wrist, and then shove another one into your leg or arm, depending on which nerves they are testing. Then they would wiggle the top needle around until a speaker made these guttural sounds. The tests went on for a few hours, until I finally said, "Enough!" I knew what was going on — I was being used as a test dummy at the Mayo Clinic and did not appreciate it one bit. Finally, after three days, I was told that I was fucked. This isn't necessarily a medical term, but it does suffice under these conditions. That was my second opinion.

Around the same time, a friend of mine needed money. He approached me and asked if I wanted to buy a .38 Special, snub-nose revolver. He said that it came from the Pagan motorcycle gang and was a "killer" gun, meaning that someone used it to kill someone. I bought it! The thing was loaded with "Dum Dum" bullets. These have a hole in them so that when they hit you, the lead blows apart and does maximum damage to your soft tissue. I kept that gun wrapped up in an old towel, under the couch cushion in the living room. Late at night, after a few mind-numbing leg spasms, I would sit there playing with this gun, taking the shells out, wiping everything off, testing the "action" and "trigger pull" and just basically trying to convince myself to put it on my forehead and pull the trigger. I was seriously thinking about taking myself out because I had lost hope. I couldn't see an end to this misery — so why not just end it?

As a little footnote to this suicide story, something happened — or, I should say, *didn't* happen — that begs to be said. I drank myself into alcoholism, mainly because of two things: Vietnam and chronic pain. I would not suggest this form of self-pain control, because the cure is just as bad, obviously, as the symptoms. It required eight years for me to finally get sober. I don't really like breaking my own confidentiality like this, but it is important for this part of the story. I have been sober for more 34 years, and I attribute that success to my involvement in Alcoholics Anonymous. This entire episode involving the gun under the cushion went on for about two months. Here I was, thinking about blowing my head off and leaving my poor wife with a mess to clean up, not to mention her not receiving any insurance money. Several months after all of this quieted down, I was at an AA meeting when it suddenly occurred to me that I never thought about *drinking* as a form of pain relief. It would have been a lot easier just to go out and buy a half gallon of vodka and drink myself to death. If you think that recovery doesn't work — just try it; you may feel differently. The bottom line

The Chronicles of Pain

here is this: Chronic pain *will* drive you into alcohol abuse, especially if you start mixing pain medication with booze and if the chronic pain is ongoing; you will eventually think about offing yourself. Please, think about it before you act — there is always some kind of solution. Why fix a temporary problem with a permanent repair?!

If you want to know what happened, I will relate the story to you. For months, throughout this horrendous period in my life, I was receiving treatment at Roper Hospital in Charleston. Two doctors — a father-and-son team-ran a pain clinic there. They were injecting cocktail of drugs directly into my spinal column, trying to reduce the pain and the subsequent leg problems. One day, during the darkest hour of my suicidal thoughts, the father doctor called me. He said that they wanted to try something different. And they did.

I went into Roper Hospital and made my way up to the second floor, where Dr. Ivestor was waiting for me. He mixed up a pile of drugs and said, "I am going to inject you with every drug that has the syllable *caine* in it." The treatment worked; my pain was reduced a little, and the leg cramps started to subside.

Here is another interesting story relating to my pain-clinic experience in Charleston. Actually, I will tell you two different stories so that you will get your money's worth from this book.

I went into Roper for my regular injection. When I came out of the room with the doctors, I had to stay in a hospital bed for an hour or two, waiting for my legs to stop being numb. This was one of the side effects of spinal-column injections: Your legs go numb. So, this became standard operating procedure. Every month, they would shoot me up, and I would lie there for a few hours until I could feel my legs and walk again. Sounds scary, doesn't it? Well, desperate times require desperate measures. After playing with a .38 snub-nose revolver for more than two months, this inconvenience was a "walk in the park" (pun intended).

Doctor Ivestor called me one day and said, "Jason, come into the clinic tomorrow. We have some other ideas for dealing with your pain." So, I went in the next morning. I removed my shirt, and the good doctor and his son started to work on me. I hate when they stick that huge needle into my back; the thing gives me the heebie-jeebies — or something similar (I'm giving away my age here!).

After the procedure, I was wheeled out into the bed area, where Nurse Jackson would care for me. Naturally, I expected to be there about two hours and that it would be no big deal. After several minutes, I noticed that my legs were going numb, but the real problems started when I tried to raise my right arm to scratch my nose. I could not raise my arm. So, I tried the left one — same thing: No response. I called the nurse over and said, "Mrs. Jackson, there is something wrong. I can't feel my arms."

She went nuts. She ran into the other room and shouted for the doctors. They came barreling out and checked me over really fast. They asked me about the numbness, and I told him that I could feel only my head. They started shooting me up with all kinds of drugs to help stop this reaction. The doc went on to explain that not only had he used a different compound but injected it a little higher than he usually did. The drugs had run *up* my spinal column rather than *down*. But they caught it in time. I asked what would have happened if they hadn't. He told me that my heart and lungs would have just stopped working and that I would be on my way to meet my ancestors.

Everything was cool. I understood the principle he was explaining to me as I lay there, numbed out. After the emergency was over, everyone went back to whatever they were doing before the code blue. It was just my head, touching my pillow. That was all that I could feel — nothing else. The entire rest of my body ceased to exist. I realized that I had become a chemically induced paraplegic. At first it was interesting; I thought, *Now I can relate to the guy who played Superman in the movies, Christopher Reeves.*

But after about 10 minutes, I got scared. *What if this doesn't wear off? Damn, I'll be in a wheelchair forever, not to mention the fan mail from Stephen Hawking.* This could prove to be a really bad thing. It eventually wore off; rather than lying there for two hours, I was a guest of the pain clinic for about five hours that day. My wife was surprised when I walked into the house. "Where have you been?" she asked. I told her that I'd been thinking.

In my first book, *a. PUZZLED EXISTENCE*, I related a story about my stay in the Oakland Naval Hospital in San Francisco. To paraphrase the story, it would go like this: Every day, I had to take my meals in a cafeteria. Three times a day, I would walk down there and sit alone. It was the most horrible thing that I had to do for many a month. I was surrounded by Marines in various forms of broken bodies. There must have been at least 30 guys in that room along with their girlfriends, wives, and moms. These men were completely broken; some had both arms missing, or both legs; one guy had all of his limbs gone. Another poor bastard was missing half of his face. Every single man in there had some kind of catastrophic injury.

Please remember, I was on the river boats in

The Chronicles of Pain

Vietnam. I heard that the Viet Cong had figured something out. If they just *kill* a Marine, his buddies will look but then keep moving with guns blazing. But, if a fellow Marine is *injured*, say, with the use of a small booby trap, something just big enough to take off a leg or arm, or even half of a face, his pals will stop, grab the guy, and drag him back behind the front line. This action may take up to six Marines out of the fight, which is an advantage to the opposing forces.

I suspected that, if I'd had my standard-issue Colt .45 and a box of shells with me, the guys would have told me to lock the doors and go around putting a bullet in all of their heads. They would beg me to finish the job.

These were the type of thoughts that ran through my head while I lay there paralyzed from the neck down. Not very happy thoughts, when you think about it.

After what seemed a lifetime, I could move only a little finger, and then two; after a while, I could lift my arm. Then came my belly and my scrotum, and there it paused. I spent a few moments of reflection on the guys at the Oakland Naval Hospital. They probably placed more emphasis on the anatomical region, the scrotum area, much more than I ever did. For them, it was gone, a lump of flesh on a piece of wax paper in some deli. I spent five hours being just a head, but that head was full of thoughts from a war that had happened long ago. Those poor bastards — I wish I could go back and finish the job some Viet Cong had started in 1970.

That's enough of that. This isn't the venue for lodging those types of arguments. Let me move on to the next pain-clinic story.

A cousin of mine, Mary, lived in Charleston and had for a very long time. She knew everyone because of her nursing career in that area. Mary called me one day and told me about an inpatient clinic at Roper. It lasted 21 days and was supposed to be quite comprehensive in scope. I called my attorney and asked him if I should go there. He concurred with my cousin Mary, and, so, I went into this 21-day program.

The first thing that I noticed was the erratic meal schedule. The food came in these big, black, plastic hot cases and was sometimes cold. It turns out that this "pain clinic" had a contract with the hospital to provide food. But it went much deeper than that. These pain people were not really affiliated with the hospital at all — they simply rented space in their other building, the one the hospital kept cobwebs in. I knew something was amiss from the first day. They had this small freezer chest that was full of Styrofoam cups of solid ice. This was their go-to method of dealing with chronic

The Chronicles of Pain

pain. You had to rub the affected area until it went numb, and *Voila!* No pain. The problem was, I knew a lot about numb body parts from a previous experience. So, time passed with a daily regimen of physical therapy, cups of ice, and bad food.

After about a week or so, a really strong pain started in the left side of my back. This was different from my usual pain — it was a burning sensation. Each day, it seemed to get worse. I mentioned this to the counselor and asked to be taken for an X-ray. It never happened. There were only two people running this entire show — the director and his right-hand man, the purveyor of ice cups. Every other day I mentioned this increasing hot, burning pain in my back, and they would hand me another chunk of ice. This went on for the entire two weeks remaining in this program.

After I got out, I flew up to Scranton, Pennsylvania, and spoke to my regular neurosurgeon, Dr. Black. He admitted me into the CMC hospital and ordered an X-ray. The next day, I was in the operating room having a tumor the size of a baseball removed from my back. He told me what it was. It had a long medical name that I couldn't pronounce, let alone remember. Black told me that these are not that uncommon and that they grow out of the nerves in one's back. All I knew was it left a big hole there, and I was on a vacuum pump for more than a week in that hospital. At least the food was hot.

There is a funny story in my book *Urban Gothic*[2] about what happened when I returned to Charleston and made it a point to go visit my super-duper pain-clinic people and explain what they had missed completely.

Several years passed, and, one day, I received a newspaper clipping from my cousin Mary. In that news article, they explained that the "pain clinic" I'd spent 21 days at — during which I was in dire pain for more than 14 of those days — *had been a complete fraud.* The two guys who operated it were being sought; they had skipped town with all of that insurance money that they'd conned from people like me — desperate people in chronic pain who will try anything to get some relief.

They were eventually caught and sent to prison. The cheeky bastards — those guys deserved every day they spent behind bars. It never fails to amaze me how people can capitalize on another person's misery, especially when that individual is in dire pain. But money is money, and we live in a society where some will do anything to acquire more

---

[2] *Urban Gothic* is a volume — actually, there are two volumes — of adult-themed short stories of a very humorous type. If you need a good laugh, go ahead and get a copy of the book.

of it.

With that said, allow me to move on to the next chapter, which deals with drugs (pain medications), therapies, and devices.

Chapter 2

Drugs, Therapies, and Devices

Most of the time, a Primary Care Physician (PCP) would prescribe a pile of Vicodin. I started my career with Darvon "pearls" diluted in a can of beer and then went on to codeine in the form of Tylenol 3s and 4s. The number denotes the amount of codeine in the formula. I then moved onto Vicodin, or as it is known by its formulaic name, hydrocodone in an acetaminophen base.

Whenever you use these opiate medications, be prepared for some really crazy dreams. This isn't the only side effect to this compound — I'll get to that later in this chapter — but it is one of those that are not often talked about. Your dreams are also in color — can you imagine that? Wild dream rides in technocolor! There are a few other pain medications available, but these are the ones I have had the most experience within my own life. One drug that has completely devastated the state of West Virginia — Oxycodone — used to come in the family of Percodan and Percocet, but, now, it's sold under its original name, Oxycodone. "Purdue Pharma" is responsible for this drug — one of the more insidious pain medications. That family of drugs includes Oxycontin and Dilaudid, both of which, given the chance, will kill you.

Going back as far as the 1980s, the medical

community decided that no one should have to endure severe pain. If a common aspirin or some other analgesic which you could buy over the counter (OTC) didn't curb the pain, they would prescribe a strong medication, usually in the form of an opioid. In the previous chapter, I alluded to the "Pain Assessment Scale." At this juncture, I am going to go into a little more detail about that unit of measurement and provide you with the actual definitions applicable to each specific number. Here is the introduction to the infamous "Smiley Face/ Pain Assessment" chart. On one end, starting with "0," there is a smile on our little round friend; this signifies no pain. On the other end, represented by a grimace — more or less a vile frown with tears streaming down the little round race — is a number "10," which signifies "Worst Possible" pain.

You then had four in between, showing various levels of pain. A nurse or doctor would ask you to apply a numerical value to your pain level. If you told them you were at the 10 level, they would admit you into the hospital and put a morphine drip in your arm. I am exaggerating that a bit — usually the "10" answer would produce a prescription pad with a signature and DEA number on it. The level 10 is described as: "Unconscious; pain that makes you pass out." A number 6 would be: "Can't be ignored but still can work. Strong pain medications help for 3 to 4 hours." Usually, people will say "5" or "6" — I know that I was in that area. After some of my surgeries, I would be in the number 9 category: "Unable to speak. Crying out or moaning." Migraine headaches would fall under the number 8, "Activity limited a lot; can read and talk with effort, nausea, and dizziness." That sums up the old 0 to 10 pain-assessment found taped to the walls of emergency rooms and doctors' offices.

I can't really say that this numerical system of pain management applies anymore. A "Bell Curve" is a statistical device used to chart behavior and various trends. It consists of a line drawing, with scales on both top and bottom, representing either time passage, age group, or just about any other parameter that you set out to chart. Well, the curve has swung back to *not* prescribing pain medications with gusto. Now you have to ask your doctor if he thinks that they will help with your pain issues. He then will go into a diatribe about the fear of total addiction. Within one week, you would be selling your body for a couple of Vicodin. Again, I just made that up, but the abuse of these very effective pain remedies has given them a very dark reputation, due to rampant over-prescribing throughout the United States. Companies like Purdue Pharma have flooded the market in certain areas, mainly rust-belt states, where there is a higher proportion of blue-collar, difficult, and dangerous jobs.

The trouble in West Virginia started with the coal miners. My father was a coal miner in Wilkes-Barre, Pennsylvania, when I was very young. He wasn't prescribed opioid medications back then, but he still suffered from the effects of his job. I recently saw an article on YouTube concerning the deluge of opioid medications dumped into West Virginia. They claimed that there were enough pills in that state at any given time to supply every man, woman, and child with more than 400 pills each! That, my friend, happens to be a lot of morphine. There is no doubt as to the addictive qualities of this family of medication. If you consume enough of these over a period of time, chances are you will have difficulty stopping. But used as directed, for a shorter time period, these compounds prove to be an effective pain-control mechanism.

Well, what *is* "a short period of time"? In my experience, it is usually one week — two weeks, maximum, if the pain persists. Anything longer than that will have consequences when it comes time to quit. You may not get "Dope Sick," as some addicts do, but you will sweat a lot, get confused, and find yourself somewhere else in your personality. It won't be pleasant, but it will last only a few days at most. Continued use and/or abuse leads to becoming "Dope Sick" during withdrawal. This condition has certain symptoms. It starts with severe joint pain, preceded or followed by profuse sweating and the sensation of hot and cold bodily feelings. Believe it or not, you also get diarrhea, a considerable amount of diarrhea, so stay close to your "Thunder Mug," as they call it in Ireland! It doesn't stop there. There will be sleeplessness and confusion, a feeling of desperation, and an overpowering desire to get more drugs at any cost. This is what addicts call being "Dope Sick."

Some people mediate this situation by using just enough medication to keep them slightly above the Dope Sickness but not actually *high*. This is called a "maintenance schedule."

Speaking of getting high, it has been my experience that when you are taking these medications for real pain, you don't get high, strictly speaking. At least that has been my observation. But there are a few other morphine-based medications out there that should be approached with caution. One of those is called "Fentanyl."

Fentanyl, a product of "Janssen Pharmaceuticals," was developed for use as a transdermal Duragesic. It is mainly found in the form of a subcutaneous, i.e., beneath the skin, patch that adheres to the skin surface. The drug then enters the body in measured doses through a specially developed membrane on the patch itself. When first introduced, this drug came in a variety of dosages: 12 mg, 25 mg, 50 mg, 75 mg, and the highest, 100 mg. The 100 mg patches are a pretty decent size. I know that, when I was placed on this medication, there were two things that stood out. The first was having to buy a clear plastic patch to place over the Fentanyl so that it didn't fall off during periods of sweaty activity or when taking a shower. The other problem that I had was the development of an extreme rash under the patch. I don't know if you've ever used a "Zippo" cigarette lighter or not, but when you filled one of those with lighter fluid and shoved it into your pocket, you would develop a stinging, itchy sore the same shape as the lighter itself.

That is what these Fentanyl patches did to me. They left rectangular areas all over my chest and back where the patch had been. These sores were very painful and required a few days to heal. Just think about it: the 100 mg size patch left an area of sheer discomfort about 1½ inches x 3 inches on your skin. It turned out that I was allergic to the adhesive used on the patch, not so much the medication itself. It got to the point where my wife would say, "You don't have any clear areas left to stick these things on!"

Because they are a transdermal system, you have to be careful how you handle the patch. If you use your fingers too much in applying the patch, the drug will enter through the skin on your fingers also. There was another drawback to using the Fentanyl Transdermal system: The effects didn't last as long as they were supposed to. The instructions would say that each patch would be sufficient for approximately three days. I never got more than two days out of the 100 mg size application.

The delivery of the pain medication had a distinct curve to it. When you first applied the thing, you would get relief very quickly; then, by the second day, you could feel the effects wearing off. This presented a dilemma: Each patch was supposed to be good for three days, but, by the third day, I wouldn't be getting any relief at all. This would lead to an overuse of the medication, which caused dire problems when you went to get a refill. Ten patches were supposed to last one month; they rarely prescribed more than that, and the stuff wouldn't last 30 days! And, since the delivery system was a patch, there wasn't any way for you to abuse this drug. So, it wasn't a fault of the patient — the problem was in the system itself.

Fentanyl killed a lot of medical students when it first came out. The Duragesic Fentanyl is considered to be at least 10 times as strong as regular morphine. You can see the liquid inside the patch; before you removed the backing, you could push it around with your fingers — it was that obvious. These med students were using a hypodermic needle to extract the contents from the patch and then injecting it. Early on, this led to overdosing and subsequent death, due to the enhanced strength of the drug.

Fentanyl is an opioid-based medication, similar to morphine, hydromorphine, methadone, oxycodone, and oxymorphine. It is a dangerous drug that should *never* — I repeat, *never* — be mixed with alcohol. You even have to be careful operating a car or heavy machinery of any sort, due to the suppressed reaction and drowsiness that it causes. Go ahead — ask me how I know so much about these pain medications. The answer to that question is a given — I used them all. I had to stop using this drug completely, not only due to the rashes all over my body, but also because I operated heavy equipment for a living. The two did not mix; I became dangerous on the job, and others noticed it.

Please keep in mind that it was never my intention to *get high*. I had a very high security clearance and worked on job sites for the

The Chronicles of Pain

federal government in both Boulder, Colorado (Rocky Flats), and in Key West, Florida, at the Naval Air Station (NAS) on Stock Island. Also, there was the Coast Guard Station in downtown Key West, where they brought in all of the contraband drugs, usually in shot-up boats. At that time, no one was giving me money not to work; in order to live and exist in these places, I didn't have much of a choice. Plus, I'll tell you this: I didn't *want* to get high. That wasn't my intention; I needed to quell the pain level just enough to allow me some semblance of normalcy. I needed to be able to walk among the living without staggering and talk without slurring my words. A number of laborers' lives depended on me operating that machine with proficiency. These guys would be 15 feet in the ground while I swung huge pipes over their heads and into place. Would you go down into a trench with some messed-up backhoe operator above your head?

Finally, I had outlived the usefulness of pill- or patch-based pain medications. After the Vicodin, Lortab, codeine, and Fentanyl patches, I progressed to a morphine pump. This thing was something else. I am not talking about the type they use in hospitals with the push-button measured dose. I'm referring to the type that is subcutaneously delivered — implanted under your skin. It's refilled once a month (or thereabouts), using a hypodermic needle. They would sometimes tattoo your site so as to know where to inject the refill, or "mother ship" arrival.

The story about this morphine pump and its installation is a juicy one that deals with fraud, deceit, and the allure of the almighty dollar!

For one of my back surgeries at CMC hospital in Scranton, Pennsylvania, I think it was in 1984 or 85, I was attended by an Indian doctor who assisted the anesthesiologist. I am not at liberty to use his name, but let's just refer to him as "Patel." After this particular surgery, number five, I was still in serious pain. Dr. Patel came to me and said that he had been working on a procedure which promised to melt the scar tissue in my back. This technique consisted of drilling a hole in the coccyx, at the base of the vertebrae terminus in the spinal column. He then injected a concoction of drugs of his own design into a catheter. These drugs did two things: they made you nauseous, and they made you itch. Your entire body would itch like crazy, everywhere, at the same time. So, Patel would inject me full of more drugs to deal with the itchiness and extreme nausea.

I lived in Charleston, South Carolina, at the time. Every month I would fly up to Scranton, Pennsylvania, take a cab to the hospital, check in for a week, and undergo this experimental

The Chronicles of Pain

treatment. I made this trip five times! The treatment did not work. Chalk up another one to medical science.

So, the same guy, Dr. Patel, decided that my best option was to have a subcutaneous morphine pump installed and that he was just the man to do the job. Teresa was with me when we met with this guy. He showed us this really slick little pump thing, about the size of a ladies' compact, weighing almost nothing. So, I said, "OK, I'll go through with this procedure." Before this, Patel had been prescribing me all kinds of opiate-based pain pills and decided that the feds were getting a little too close for comfort (I'll explain the reason why shortly). So, he put the morphine pump in, just to the right of my lower stomach. When I came out of surgery, I felt this huge mass of iron in my stomach. When the doctor came into my room, I said, "What the hell is this, doc? This thing feels like a lump of pig iron. What happened to the slick little thing you showed us?" He rubbed his chin a bit and looked around before answering.

Patel went on to say that when he finally did the surgery, lo and behold, there weren't any of those newer type pumps on the shelf, so he had to use this older one. In the textile business, this is usually referred to as the "bait and switch" technique. Pitch a big sale with brand-name designer clothes, and then substitute some cheaper variety. I began to suspect that something was not quite right, but what was my recourse? I had this giant hole in my belly that just happened to be filled with a miniature scrap yard, so I kept the damn thing in.

This was at the beginning of the summer, and I was helping my brothers in the family excavating business, driving a big truck. Needless to say, this doctor from India failed to tell me that the pump operated on body heat: The more heated up I got, the more morphine it pumped into my back area. But the terminus of the pipeline to my back was just shoved in there, between two vertebrae, so this drug was basically being pumped directly into my entire body. The result was quite predictable — I started to get high as a kite, not the state to be in when you're barreling down a highway with 20 tons of stone pushing you along. I had to quit the job, and this left my brothers high and dry — no pun intended.

Another thing about this damn pump was that it made me completely impotent. It didn't matter what my wife tried; nothing was working. My willie had simply gone out on strike. I didn't know Patel was a teamster! So, the outcome of this fiasco was apparent. I had him rip the thing out of my body, and old Patel wasn't too happy about that, because he was being paid a princely sum to refill it every month. On the day of the surgery, his partner in crime, as it turned out, really poured on the gas to knock me out cold. I felt and tasted the result of that surgery for a week, and a feeling of complete "pathos" settled in on me. It was an unnerving sensation I hope never to feel again. A case of excess anesthesia if there ever was one.

As it turned out, this character Patel and his trusty sidekick, "Gasman," were charged with insurance fraud. They installed these inferior pumps, always at the last minute. Do you think for one minute that a doctor would go into the operating room without all of the parts he would need to complete the surgery? They were charging the insurance companies the full markup on one of those slick, designer morphine pumps — and then installing an old clunker. The VA always sent me the bills for my file. That particular surgery cost a little more than $86,000, *and* they charged the VA to remove the bastard. Before these bums could be brought to justice, they skipped town and returned to India. How fitting it was when, afterward, the authorities looked into these two individuals more closely, it was discovered that they had forged credentials. Now *that's* rich!

This was the second time that I had been bamboozled by fake medical personnel, and both times, my pain levels increased, because *after they removed the pump, they wouldn't answer my calls.* My only hope is that, someday, I will run into Dr. Patel and his stooge in a dark alley somewhere. I would need just enough time to remove their kidneys so that I could donate them to someone on the black market who needs a few.

There is a simple idiom that has served me well over the years, and I would like to explain it to you. Here is how I look at the use of narcotic pain medications in my life. The lack of these medications will compromise the quality of my life far more than the supposed stigma of addiction. To put this into simpler terms, allow me to say this: Taking a controlled substance to quiet severe pain is far superior to having a gun placed on your forehead.

If you recall, earlier in this book, I related the story about a 21-day inpatient pain clinic that turned out to be bogus. You will have to read the short story in *Urban Gothic* for the full account of that little incident. There was one important thing those gentlemen left me with. One afternoon, the guy who was in charge of the ice-cup therapy said this: "Jason, you must *own* your pain; it is yours, and no one can take it away, especially the people who care for you. As you make your displeasure known, you inadvertently render your wife, mother,

The Chronicles of Pain

girlfriend, or significant other impotent. As much as they want to try, there is absolutely nothing they can do to ease your suffering, and that is a terrible place for any meaningful person to be. Own your pain, and provide relief to those who love you…" He went on to talk about a number of other things, like telling your doctor how bad your pain level is and the need to seek out a treatment that will fit your lifestyle while controlling the pain at the same time. I can't tell you that I chiseled the words "OWN YOUR PAIN" into a large block of granite, but I did adopt this philosophy, and I use it every day of my life. Not too many people know that I live in chronic pain, primarily because I don't tell them. My wife can see it on my face, and, when that happens, I don't deny it, but I don't go on and on about it, either. It's mine, all mine — I bought and paid for it, I own it outright, and that is the way it will stay until the day I get to sleep somewhere without this constant companion.

In this chapter, I can't stress more strongly the fact that I am *not* a doctor, nor am I a pharmacist. My position is that of an individual who has gone through more surgeries, and the related pain they caused, than anyone else that I happen to know. My purpose is to tell you the details of my experience with everything that is relevant to living with chronic, unremitting pain. I just wanted to take this opportunity to reiterate my stance on these issues and their effect on one's life. With that said, allow me to move on and travel to a different realm.

My involvement with pain and the pursuit of pain reduction has spanned a total of 44 years to date. During that time, I have been exposed to a bewildering assortment of both medication-based therapies and non-invasive techniques. I am going to include an overview of some of the disciplines that I have had personal experience with. Embarking on this diversion from pharmaceuticals in a chapter about drugs seemed like the logical thing to do. By now, many of you may be asking, *What if I don't want to use* any *drugs?* And that is a valid concern.

The gamut of techniques that I have been exposed to includes: Hypnosis, acupuncture, bio-feedback, meditation, and TENS units. I will undoubtedly think of a few others before this chapter is done, but we will deal with those as they present themselves.

Let me start with the TENS units. The acronym TENS stands for **T**ranscutaneous **E**lectrical **N**erve **S**timulation. To put this into layman's terms, let me describe TENS this way: Faking the brain from sending pain mail to the rest of your body. The unit itself is quite small — a little black box that takes a 9-volt battery. There are four wire leads coming out of the box that attach to small, round sticky things you place on your area of pain. There is a set procedure for that placement, which I won't go into here, because it varies for different parts of the body. For me, it was always my back — the L4, L5, S1, S2 lower-back region. So, my stick-'em ups were pretty straightforward — a square box with the round electrodes set on each corner. Plus, there is a left and a right, so you would put a red and a black on the top corners and then put the same red-and-black configuration on the bottom corners.

Then you turn the thing on. It is a weird thing to describe, the sensation that you experience from the site. It's sort of a buzzing vibration that almost tickles, but it is pointed at the same time. I'm not doing a very good job of describing this to you, am I? Well, it's difficult, because it is a feeling unto itself. Once you experience a TENS unit, you will always be able to identify it in any future setting. A TENS unit has its own profile. But I can say this: They *work* — at least for a little while, anyway. I wore a TENS every day for two solid years. My wife would stick the little pads on my back. I would then wrap up the excess wire and tie it off with a twisty, turn the thing on, and slip it into my pocket. It kept the pain at bay, but I had to keep increasing the juice to achieve the same desired results until the day came when there wasn't any more power — like Scotty, from the *Star Trek* series, telling Captain Kirk: *"I can't get you any more power, Captain!"* How's *that* for a slight-diversion-from-a-diversion for you!

Here's another story that involves the TENS unit. After one of my back surgeries, Dr. Black installed a TENS right under the dressing on my back. It was arranged on both sides of the incision in a perfect square pattern. A day or two after the surgery, one of the nicest nurses, a sweet girl named "Joy," came in to change my dressings. I didn't realize it at the time, but I had that TENS cranked all the way up to maximum power. My body had become acclimated to the effect of the TENS after the two years of wearing one, as I mentioned in the account above. Well, she started to remove the bandage, and I heard a loud *thud!* When I asked for Joy, there was no response. I turned around, and there was Joy, flat on the floor. She had been blown out against the wall and then just slid down onto the floor. That was an example of the power of that little black box called TENS. The device would take the juice from the 9-volt battery and amplify it over and over again until it reached a phenomenal level of power. Needless to say, I felt both bad and embarrassed at the same time because it was

The Chronicles of Pain

my fault. I should have mentioned that the TENS was on. Joy survived, but she didn't like me very much after that little stunt.

Now let me tell you about meditation. Just a few miles outside the little town of Honesdale, Pennsylvania, there is a facility known as the "Himalayan Institute." As the name implies, they deal in everything from that part of the world. The school was established by the late Swami Rama, who started building a hospital at the foot of the Himalayan Mountains and then went on to found schools in various parts of the United States. I know that there is one in Chicago, and I think there is another on the west coast, in Los Angeles. You will have to Google the rest. At the "Institute" in Honesdale, they offer degree programs in a variety of subjects. If I am not mistaken, they go all the way up to a Master's Degree level. Many individuals go there to pursue studies in holistic methods for dealing with medicine, pharmaceuticals (meaning natural remedies, of course), and vegan dietary requirements and preparation. I went there to study meditation.

The Swami Rama was the guy who stopped his heart on television back in the 1960s. He slowed his heart rate to such a low point that the instruments of the day could not detect it, and he kept it that way for more than 15 minutes. He used nothing but meditation to accomplish this feat. I was fortunate enough to meet this gentleman in person during one of my trips to the Institute. In just meeting this man, you could feel the guy's aura; it was a memorable occasion, to say the least.

I enrolled in one of their condensed courses on meditation. In the space of four days, I was introduced to a number of techniques that would allow me to control my body and, more importantly, its reaction to pain. The stuff worked — as long as I practiced the methods on a daily basis, I could control my pain levels. Why I drifted away from this, I will never know. It was one of those life-changing things, but working, making a lot of money, that sort of thing filled my daily schedule to the point of not having enough time left for meditation. Work became my meditation, and cash substituted for harmony and peace. But an interesting thing occurred right after my introduction to the Himalayan Institute.

My doctors sent me to a "bio-feedback" place in Wilkes-Barre, Pennsylvania. I'm not absolutely sure what this had to do with anything at the time, but it dealt with biometrics and things of that nature. This encounter occurred right after I returned from the Himalayan Institute, and I was still practicing meditation.

What I remember of this visit was that a technician hooked me up to all of these machines. He placed a cap on my head that was filled with wires and cups with gooey stuff on them. After all of this preparation work was done, he told me to relax, close my eyes, and allow my body to just drift out into space somewhere. So, I did that — I relaxed and went to visit some of my distant relatives in another dimension. (I couldn't resist that little departure from the school course.) Anyway, they used a technique where they would place your fingers in both hot and cold water. One was really hot, and the other had ice in it, so it was really cold. During these experiments, the machine kept spitting out a continuous stream of paper with black lines on it. What I did was place myself in a meditative state commonly referred to as a "7-minute meditation."

After all of the calculations came in, the technician said to me, "This is incredible — you did not respond to any of the 'immersion' studies that I performed. Your reactions were almost completely flat!" I suspected that I should have jumped when they placed my fingers in either the hot or cold water, and I didn't. One thing I do remember is debating whether to tell them about using meditation during the entire exercise. You will have to excuse me on the lack of details concerning this encounter. I think I had only two sessions with these people, and it was a long time ago. My purpose for bringing it up was to explain some of the various techniques that I was exposed to and that are out there. You will have to decide which ones might be best for you, because every person is different when it comes to some of this science. Here are a few others:

Hydrotherapy — For this, you are going to need access to a "lap" pool. These are usually found in a decent recreation center or complete health facility. The process is fairly basic; it consists of walking in a swimming pool, holding a Styrofoam board in front of you. This may sound relatively easy, but it actually isn't — water does provide plenty of resistance. Hopefully, you will have the benefit of a good trainer —someone who knows how to deal with chronic-pain clients. The board that is used is sometimes called a "Boogie" board, patterned after a small surfboard. What you do is walk "laps" in the pool. Hydrotherapy has the added advantage of buoyancy. This helps keep the weight off of your spinal column and makes the exercise a little easier to digest, or tolerate, if you will.

Exercise is the key. It doesn't matter what age you are — a good exercise program will benefit any chronic-pain sufferer. I have been working out in gyms for many more years than I care to remember. I will probably mention this again, because exercise is really important.

The Chronicles of Pain

Acupuncture — My doctor — and the insurance company paying the bills — thought that I could benefit from having a number of acupuncture sessions. So, I went. There were 12 visits in total. The cost? $250 a shot. This guy would stick dozens of needles into my flesh and light a couple of them with a match. I would just lie there for about an hour, the standard length of a visit, and relax on a nice, soft table. Sometimes when I got home, my wife would find needles sticking out of me in rather awkward places. I guessed that he put so many in that he couldn't remember where they all were. None of this hurt; if you do experience pain, you have to tell the practitioner straightaway. If the needles are placed in the correct spots, you won't feel anything. I had a few occasions when I went off the table after the guy, but they were rare.

Here is what happened to my experiment with the world of acupuncture. Nothing! That's right —nothing happened. I didn't feel any loss of pain or any noticeable reduction in the same. There was a reason. Several months after my treatment in Wilkes-Barre, Pennsylvania, I found myself back in Charleston, South Carolina. While there, I contacted a real Chinese practitioner of acupuncture. The other guy was actually a Jewish doctor. A telephone consultation was arranged with Dr. Skeleton —

I kid you not: That was actually his name — *Skeleton*. During this conversation, the doctor asked me a pointed question: "Did you have surgery on your lower back?" So, I told him about the seven surgeries that I'd had to date and about their impact on my pain levels. He stopped me and said, "Acupuncture will not work on you because of the scar tissue blocking the pathways."

He used a technical term, but the message was quite clear. I was fucked as far as Chinese medicine was concerned. I asked him why the other guy didn't say anything about this. His reply was basically, "Kid, do I have to explain?" Naturally, it was about the money. $250 a crack times 12 visits will put a few tires on a doctor's Porsche or pay for his golf game for an entire season. The lesson here is not really a lesson at all: Sometimes it doesn't pay to have comprehensive, pay-for-everything insurance. You turn into a golden goose or some giant heifer just dying to be milked. Have I mooed yet today?

Well, I hate to say this, but there is more. I was sent for **Hypnosis**. Don't worry — this part of the conversation will be short. I went to see a guy who said he was going to hypnotize me out of pain. Let me just say this: I was in pain then, and I'm still in pain now. The hypnotist went on to explain that I wasn't a good subject for this ancient art. Fortunately, he didn't ask me for my star sign. If he had, I would have known that I was in California!

That pretty much sums up my experiences with alternative therapies that don't involve narcotic drugs. There were a few others, like wearing a piece of copper in a special belt on my lower back — that didn't end well, either. They tried to talk me into buying a mattress that was embedded with copper and crystals. I passed on that, also.

Personally, I see nothing wrong with using opioid medications to control severe, chronic pain. It's there — why not use it? That is an American philosophy — *Pragmatism*. I kid you not: Pragmatism is seen in American culture as a branch of philosophy. The best example that I know of is the sugar bowl. We Americans put two handles on it because it just made sense — and that, basically, is the definition of pragmatism. But if you are going down the path of opioid medications, there are a few things to be aware of.

One thing to remember is this: After taking the pills for a few days, and you start to get some relief, don't stop taking the medication. That is how it works. Another thing is not to drink when you are on narcotics — or you will slide sideways. If you do this, it won't turn out well. Then there is the question of gradation.

Do not stop taking pain medication abruptly; it will not make you feel happy. These compounds do build up in your system, and they can be dangerous. Reduce your dosage little by little, over a period of several days, or even weeks. This will depend on the number of opioids you have taken, and over what period of time. If you decide to stop taking these things, call your doctor first and tell him. Be honest so that he knows exactly what he is dealing with. Don't downplay the amount, because that will come back to bite you when least expected. If you do decide to ignore the label's or my warning about drinking while taking narcotics, let me just say this one last thing: Watch your head when it hits the floor.

In summary: I told you straightaway that I was neither a doctor nor a pharmacist. My entire life in dealing with chronic pain comes down to experience. I have tried just about everything to stop this clawing in my brain, the moaning, the cursing at inanimate objects (like getting out of a car), even waking up in the morning — just about anything that makes the situation worse. No — check that last word: Not worse, *known*! Something that makes the situation known: That is a better way to describe living with chronic pain — just knowing about it on a daily basis. There are new therapies involving cannabis-derived compounds. I don't know anything about these things. I never had any experience with them and probably never will. There is a very expensive reason why I used the term "never" in the last statement. I may go into detail later on in this book about the choice of words, but I can't promise anything at this time.

While I was living in Charleston, I went to see an orthopedic group. After extensive testing, they decided to install *Harrington Rods* into my back. *What are these things?* you may ask. They are two stainless steel rods — in my case, about nine inches long. They are bolted to the coccyx and extend as high as they have to go — in my case, the L-4 vertebrae. Well, they started to draw blood for this procedure in advance, which should say something about the severity of this surgery. But my wife wasn't convinced that this was the way to go and begged me to get a second opinion. I flew up to Scranton and met with Dr. Holla. This was my first encounter with the Zen surgeon. As I sat in his office asking a lot of questions, he suddenly threw a ballpoint pen on the floor at my feet and said, "Pick that up!" I thought to myself, *Pick that thing up yourself — it's your pen.* But having been raised with respect and by a very large father who thought nothing of kicking my ass in a situation like this, I got up, bent down, picked up the pen, and presented it to the good doctor with a smile. "Here's your pen, Doc."

After I sat back down, Dr. Holla said to me, "Do you see what you have just done? Well, if you have these rods put into your body, you won't be able to do that." I looked at the floor and then at him. I said, "The doctors in Charleston told me that I would have full motion after these Harrington Rods were installed!" I said this as if I were defending their honor or something as in; *What do you mean? Impossible!* Holla then told me that he takes a set of those out almost every month. He went on to explain how they loosen over time, how they restrict your range of motion, etc., etc. I then asked the same stupid question that I've used before when astonished: "Why would they tell me I would have a full range of motion after they were installed?" He just looked at me and said, "Kid, do I have to spell it out for you?" It required a moment for the truth to set in, but eventually I realized what he was saying. It was all about the money, again!

The Chronicles of Pain

Chapter Three

Backless Gowns, Bad Beds, and Jello

The Chronicles of Pain

There are generally three ways to enter a hospital. The first is you walk in under your own power. Secondly, they wheel you in, using a wheelchair driven by a "Transporter." And lastly, you are carried in through the emergency room. When this happens, words like "Stat!" and "Code Blue!" come into play, and that is not good for you, the patient. This usually means that you are in pretty bad shape. But there is one universal idiom that applies to whatever means by which you enter the facility. *Park your dignity at the front door.* I'm serious. If there is anything I have learned about entering hospitals, it is this: You do not own your own dignity after you cross that threshold.

The first thing that they do is have you undress from wearing perfectly good clothes and put on a gown that they provide which doesn't have any back to it. What happens is that you forfeit your own body to the care of the staff. They will poke and prod you in places you are rarely touched that way. They will roll you around, flop you into beds, and then transfer you to another apparatus with wheels. You will notice that just about everything you see will have wheels on it. This fact may challenge your idea of permanence. The thought occurs to you that when you wake up, you could be wheeled into the next county — or worse, a gated community made entirely of gold!

The night before a major surgery is always entertaining, unless you are unconscious, which is sometimes preferable to being awake. A parade of doctors will enter your room and introduce themselves. Then, they proceed to tell you what they are going to do to your body. I had an anesthesiologist come in one night and tell me that he was going to pump every drug that ended in "*caine*" into my body. Most of these medications will render you on a trip to Disneyland without leaving your bed. If you are unfortunate to have had multiple surgeries, such as I have, the doctors will start rattling off percentages. These are always heartwarming. My surgeon will say something along these lines: *"You realize that you have a 40% chance of not being able to poop again."* Here are a few other good ones: *"There is a possibility that you may not walk again, or you may have difficulty walking. And then there is the chance that you may never get an erection again."* Of course, all of these predictions come with their own caveats in the form of numerical percentages. *"There is a 30% chance you will come down with Hong Kong Dong." "Medicine isn't an exact science, so there is also a 60% chance that we will end up in court for a vicious battle over medical malpractice...."*

Naturally, these are extreme examples. Because I have had *so many* major surgeries,

The Chronicles of Pain

I have to go through this every time. But the worst part is when they whip out a little black thing with an ink pen attached to it with wire (so that you can't steal *their* pen), and this is where you sign all of your rights away. I'm not suggesting that you have your attorney lying in the bed next to you for the duration, but there are very real considerations to take into account. Allow me to give you an example based on my experience. This story involves my fourth back surgery, that was performed in 1988 at CMC hospital in Scranton, Pennsylvania. It was supposed to be a standard in-and-out laminectomy, but the procedure was far from the utopia they described to me.

If you recall, I mentioned the wheels you see *on everything* in a hospital. The reason for that is that you end up being wheeled all over the place. You become a connoisseur of dropped ceiling tiles and light fixtures. As they roll you into the operating room, someone with a small, round mirror on their forehead will say, "Hi," and then walk away. I had an incident once that is worth repeating. Keep in mind that you are always looking up at people's faces while lying on this stainless-steel cart. My buggy was stopped right before we went through the double doors into the operating theater. An anesthesiologist called a halt to our little procession. He said to me,

"You probably don't remember me, because I'm the guy who gives you gas that makes you fall asleep. But I wanted to take this opportunity to apologize to you for something. I always thought that you guys with back injuries were always faking it — trying to game the system or beat an insurance company out of their hard-earned money. (He laughed a little at this pun.) About a year ago, I was on the golf course and threw out my back; it turned out that I had popped a disc. Now that I know the truth, I can tell you that I have never experienced that kind of pain in my life — and I played football in college. It was mind numbing, so, I thought that, if I ever saw you again, I would make it a point to apologize to you personally. And, trust me, you will not be feeling any pain for quite a while from this procedure. I will make damn sure of that."

I was then promptly wheeled through the double doors and into the inner sanctum of the operating room. The operating room (the "OR") is like the beating heart of the hospital. First of all, they keep those places as cold as ice, so your toes will be freezing. If a nurse offers you a heated blanket, take it — don't even think about it. *Just say, "Yes."* You may have never even thought about what kind of music the surgeon likes to play while he is slicing and dicing. I don't know how important a question like that

The Chronicles of Pain

is, but, for me, it was comforting to know that my guy liked both Oldies *and* Chopin. In a perverse way, it may tell you something about your man or woman, or at least give you a touch of comfort in knowing that the person has good taste. Look at it this way: If the surgeon is into Heavy Metal, then consider yourself screwed. Nothing is going to go well on that operating table. There will be too much headbanging and use of the word "Dude."

Another little suggestion is to relax as much as possible. They are going to ask for one — or both — of your arms. Your arms will be extended onto these special little paddle things and taped there. This isn't to stop you from belting the guy cutting into you. It's for the purpose of sticking needles into your arms for various condiments, small bags of weird-looking stuff that they pump into you during the procedure.

Another thing: Remember the idiom at the start of this chapter? The one about parking your dignity at the door? Well, it applies here, also. Don't waste any time or thought about a bunch of people staring at your private parts. They have seen it all before, and nothing, aside from another appendage growing out of your belly, is going to alarm them. So just forget about your vanity — it doesn't apply here. You can always tell the "gas man" to give you a little something to make you completely ridiculous, but enough of that will be forthcoming anyway. When the guy tells you to count backwards from 10, do it — because you won't make it to six. I can assure you of that.

It is interesting to note that, at the VA hospital that I go to, they have hand-painted tiles in the dropped ceiling, so as they roll you down to the abattoir, you get to look at the occasional Andrew Wyeth scene — birds, snow-covered wagons, little kids frolicking by a nuclear power plant. You know, nice warm, fuzzy things of that nature. Naturally, at the VA, there are a lot of American flags and battle scenes from the Pacific theater of war. You know — tanks, guns, people getting blown to kingdom come — nice memorable thoughts while they roll you into surgery

During my (I *think*) fifth back surgery at the CMC hospital in Scranton, Pennsylvania, I experienced everything that I just told you about, went into the OR as ordered, and committed to surgery. Everything was going along just as to be expected, until I got to the PAC unit. This is the place where they watch you like a hawk as you come out of your chemically induced trip to a distant nebula. There are all kinds of wires and monitors attached to you, and there are computer screens all over the place with little black lines jumping across a white plane.

The Chronicles of Pain

The really nice nurses usually work in the PAC units, and they stop by your bed and ask you repeatedly how you feel. I mean, your head is spinning, and the grogginess resembles a Saigon whorehouse, but, other than that, you feel just ducky. Well, this time I wasn't so sure. It turns out that, during this standard lower-back surgery, someone, inadvertently, without malicious intent, nicked my spinal cord. That was the operative word — *nicked*. I asked the nurse, "What exactly does *nicked my spinal column* mean?" She told me that it means just that — they accidentally sliced my spinal column. The scalpel just slipped, sort of like a Japanese restaurant without the sushi.

The next thing that happened was I tried to move and couldn't. I asked the nurse, "Excuse me, madam. Would you be so kind as to explain to me why I cannot move?" She went on to explain, in "medicalese," why I was strapped to the bed with three huge nylon ropes. They reminded me of the harnesses they use to lift giant air-conditioning units up to the 150th floor of a new skyscraper in Shanghai. My "handler" nurse explained that I was strapped to the bed and would remain that way for an extended period of time, due to the slice in my spinal cord. My spinal fluid was leaking, and any movements could render me a wheelchair occupant for all eternity. This was really great

— just the kind of news you want to hear after spending four hours in surgery and lying in a stainless-steel environment somewhere in the bowels of the hospital.

This "incident" is the perfect introduction into the world of bedpans and catheters, not to mention the pleasant thoughts about frolicking in an Irish glade.

There are several items about the hospital experience which haven't yet been discussed in this tutorial: The *bedrails* and the *urinal*. Allow me to address the latter first. (I call the urinals "torpedoes," for some reason. Don't ask me why — it just happened that way.

The fact that I am a male allows me the benefit of knowledge concerning a torpedo's operation. As for the female version, I have seen them once or twice, but I must admit, I don't know what it's like to use a female torpedo. For that reason, I will delegate that information to the woman who writes a book of this nature. But I have had more experience with the male torpedo. Most of these things are made from plastic. I was in a hospital in San Francisco having a vasectomy; I recall that the urinals were papier-mâché composite. I'm *serious*. At first, I was waiting for the bottom to fall out of the thing, although — trust me — after you have a vasectomy, urinating is a memorable occasion.

The Chronicles of Pain

As mentioned above, urinals are mostly made from plastic. I have never turned one over to check the recycle symbols, but I'm sure hospitals recycle *everything*. One dumpster is labeled "body parts," and another has "recycle" written on it. One of the major things that I can tell you straightaway is this: There is a lip on the inside of the top part — the hole you put your little Ambrose in, if it rubs the edge, the effect could be uncomfortable. The possibility exists that you could scratch yourself "down there," and that could have serious consequences. Also, the things are designed with this bend in the "neck." It is supposed to facilitate their use while you're in a seated position. Though I wouldn't mind seeing that designer in my basement some night. When you're in a prone position, it takes some finesse to master the art of torpedo usage, and the possibility exists that you may have very wet fingers afterward. Whatever you do, don't pour your old recycled drinking water into the torpedo. You may ask why someone would do something like that, and it would be a valid question.

My reasoning is this: Men are capable of many strange behaviors. Right after your surgery, they are going to want to measure all of the liquids coming out of you. That bag hanging above your head is full of saline solution. It keeps your IV from freezing up, among other things, so what goes in must come out. Hospital personnel need to know that it's *all* coming out. Where else this liquid would go is anyone's guess but, I suppose someone will explain that later on. When I decided to write *The Chronicles of Pain*, I wanted to explore every possible avenue leading to pain and what it does to a person or — more to the point — what it does to me! The lip on the urinal can cause pain. Ask me how I know this. Or better yet, leave that question unanswered for now; we'll explore it in more detail later on. Naturally, I can attest to what a plastic scratch feels like on that sensitive part of a man's anatomy, and it's a hell of a place to put a Band-Aid!

Your urinal is usually shoved onto the infamous *rail*. There are two of these, one on each side of the bed. When you come back from the OR and the PAC unit, they will first slide you off the gurney and onto the regular bed with a *1, 2, 3, ugh* sort of motion. As soon as you hit the new bed, up go the rails, and you're locked in for the night. If you ask about the rails, a nurse will say that it's for your own protection. Those rails are very difficult to drop when you are in the bed, and if you do manage this feat, it will make a lot of noise, which will alert the nursing squad, and someone will appear, darkening your door with the question, "Mr. Goodman, are *we* going somewhere?" I

The Chronicles of Pain

usually tell them that I have this strange urge to breakdance.

The reason that I am spending any amount of time on the *rails* has to do with the *torpedoes*. Now would be a good time to say, *"Damn the torpedoes!"* Well, not exactly. First of all, it would be a bad pun, and, secondly, you're going to need that urinal. Why the rails are significant is this: It's easier to use a torpedo when your leg is hanging over the edge of the bed as opposed to lying down. Something else to keep in mind is the fact that, depending on the area where the surgery was performed, you will have to demonstrate an ability to pee before they will even talk about letting you go home. For example, remember when I mentioned "the percentages" they give you the night before the event? Well, one of those has to do with the ability to urinate. If you are having a tough time making that happen, they will want to know why. It may mean that something is wrong in the plumbing department. This could also apply to Number Two!

I don't know about you, but I try to avoid the use of bedpans at all costs. I look at it this way: If people go on hunger strikes in jails over some issue, I will go on a constipation strike to avoid the use of a bedpan. First of all, they keep them in the refrigerator. You know that I'm making that up, but that is how it feels when they slide it under your buttocks. That is a strange word — *buttocks*. It sounds like a sort of vegetable, as in, "How are the Buttocks today — are they fresh?"

Don't forget the sacred "idiom." *Thou shalt deposit your dignity, and further claim, to your being, whereas, habeas corpus included, at the front door of the designated hospital.* When it comes to bedpans, unless you are high as a kite on morphine, they can really tax anyone's resolve to maintain some form of normalcy while performing *that* particular bodily function. My advice, or suggestion, if that sounds less intimidating, is to just do it. Don't think about it; don't stress about it; put the whole experience out of your mind.

The reason I say these things is quite simple: What is your alternative when you're strapped to a bed and can raise your head only 20 degrees? A big hole in the bed would do the trick, but in all of my experience, I've never seen anything on wheels that looked like that. I will leave you with one sage word of advice: Make sure the bedpan is placed correctly. I had a guy, a male nurse (more on him later) who later confessed that he was stealing my Dilaudid injections (for post-surgical pain) and substituting saline solution. He positioned the bedpan backwards. This was my very first experience involving one of these vessels, and

The Chronicles of Pain

he fucked it up. Naturally, I did my business all over the bed and myself. Unbeknownst to me, he was high at the time, and he actually found it all very funny. If it hadn't been for the three nylon straps holding me down, I would have reduced this dude to hamburger meat if I could have gotten out of that bed. At very least, I would have had him strapped down and made to use this device for a few weeks — a little *justice karma*, as in, "My *karma* ran over my *dogma*" (hospital humor?)

Now, about that male nurse. Marty (I changed his name, even though the guy is dead) had been stealing pain medications from patients for years. I often wondered why I was in so much pain during the dayshift hours. Whenever I complained, the doctors and hospital personnel would automatically think I was just trying to get more drugs. Nurses usually think that way, especially when they get a guy like me, having had multiple surgeries, and a bit too hospital savvy for my own good. Their decision would almost automatically be: Drug searcher! AKA, someone who is always looking for more of anything with morphine in it.

So, Marty continued to work there, and I, along with a number of other patients, continued to suffer excess pain immediately after surgery. At the time, my wife, Teresa, and

I were living in Charleston. One day, Marty and his girlfriend decided to move down there. They stayed with us for a few days until they found an apartment, and they both got jobs as nurses at the local hospitals. Marty asked me to "sponsor" him in the AA program of alcohol abuse recovery, and I agreed. I won't even try to explain what a sponsor does — you'll have to look that up.

So, one night, Marty and I were cruising down this dark country road on our way to an AA meeting, and he told me that he had a confession to make. Then he went into detail about stealing my pain medications, and he was sorry, blah, blah, blah. Meanwhile, I was trying desperately to figure out how to eject him from my vehicle while driving down a paved road at 60 mph. I just wanted to watch him bounce down the road in my rearview mirrors; I would have thoroughly enjoyed every minute of his agony.

Fate has a way of taking its toll. Marty was diagnosed with HIV, the virus that results in AIDS. He claimed that it came from a bad batch of blood used to treat his hemophilia, but I think it may have come from a dirty needle. But it's a moot question because this guy died there, in Charleston. His girlfriend sold everything and moved back to Scranton without even saying "Thank you" to my wife and me. But she's okay, as there was a large life-insurance policy on my nemesis Marty for her to cash in.

It happens — drugs are stolen on a regular basis, either for personal use, as per my friend, Marty, or for selling. Some of these narcotic medications are worth a phenomenal amount of money on the street. But that is another subject entirely. We will look at that subject more in depth later in the book, but for now, I would like to stick with the subject at hand. And that is (drumroll): *catheters*!

For people of the feminine persuasion, I understand that a catheter isn't that big a deal. I honestly don't know; you would have to ask them. I did inquire of my wife once after she had some minor surgery that involved the application of that device, and she told me it wasn't too uncomfortable. I definitely cannot say that about a man, especially this man! I actually hate having to fantasize about being a pornographic movie star while they work on the insertion. I would love to hear the OR (Operating Room) people say ...*they have to send out for a much longer tube....* but that never happens. I am simply stuck with what I have down there.

Allow me to relate a little incident that occurred about a year ago. In 2019, my right leg was not getting enough blood flow below the knee, making the act of walking a very difficult endeavor. One of the issues attached to having been exposed to Agent Orange in Vietnam is what they call *ischemic heart disease*. One characteristic of this condition is developing aneurisms, and that is what happened several years ago while I was flying back from Ireland. I went right into the VA hospital in Philadelphia, and they operated on an abdominal aneurysm located in my groin area, at the top of my right leg. It turned out that the stint they'd installed had bent into a 90-degree angle, and that was inhibiting blood flow.

I checked in one morning, and by the afternoon, I was spending close to four hours on the operating table. It turned out to be a more involved procedure than the doctors had anticipated. They installed another stint, cleaned up some blood vessels that looked a little iffy, and glued me back together. I kid you not — they didn't use staples to close the exterior of the wound. They did use sutures *inside* to stitch together whatever it was they put in there, but the outside was *glued* together. I had never had this before. Granted, I have used glue on a few occasions to stick together some busted-up fingers on a job site. That's right: glue and duct tape are standard medical supplies when you're out in the woods with a bulldozer. Gasoline may be available to use as an anesthetic, but that would be a luxury.

The Chronicles of Pain

So, for this vascular surgery, they glued the wound closed and inserted a catheter. This was against my wishes, but the surgeon made it a point to tell me that he didn't want me pissing on his hands while he was working. I could accept that! They used tape to hold the tubing for the catheter to my leg. I don't know where they got this tape from, but, man, it was stuck there for good. It must have been medical-grade Gorilla tape or something, because that tube wasn't going anywhere. But therein lay the problem.

Before I relate the rest of this story, allow me to post a disclaimer. I am not bragging, nor am I a porn star, as I discussed earlier. I am simply relating a true story which actually has a medical application that every doctor should realize when they tape a catheter to a man's leg. After the PAC unit, the doc came in to see me. He told me it had gone well and that it was more screwed up than he thought. But he said that they had fixed everything and that I should be going home the next day. "You will be spending the night here, and I'll have them send up some dinner. See you in the morning!"

I was in bed. The catheter was doing all the work for me, and I didn't have to do a Number Two, so I was good. My wife brought me some food; I watched a little television and then fell asleep. Pretty uneventful. Late that night is when the trouble began. For some reason, I had developed a very large and extremely persistent nocturnal erection. To this day, I haven't a clue where this thing came from. I don't use any kind of enhancement medicine, and I wasn't looking at a centerfold — it was just one of those things. At 70 years old, I should welcome any kind of an erection, especially the nocturnal type, but there was a painful caveat to this one.

When I first awoke, I noticed a pain at the very top of my johnson; this pain kept getting more and more intense. When I finally pulled up the sheet and gave it a look, there was the tube, digging into my member. The taped tube wasn't long enough, and, as I mentioned, this tape wasn't going anywhere. So, I had to start slapping "Nuba" around to try to stop the reaction, sort of like pulling rods out of the reactor at Chernobyl. Look, I'm not trying to brag here — they just didn't leave enough slack in the pipeline to accommodate this possibility, as remote as it may have seemed. That thing hurt like *hell*, and I *did* relate the incident to my doctor the next time I saw him. My request was simple: Put a loop in — then there would room for "expansion."

I hate catheters, and this incident did nothing but intensify my negative feelings toward them. If you are having a surgery that requires the use of a catheter, make sure to tell them to leave a little slack in the pipe, just in case. Or, photocopy these pages, and have the doctor read what can happen with one small lapse in judgment — pain, especially in that particular area.

Hospital beds are not designed for comfort. They roll you up from the PAC unit and into a hospital room. There will be a lot of activity; many personnel will get involved transferring you to the regular bed. It usually goes like this — *1, 2, 3, umph,* — and three or four people slide you across from the gurney into your new home for a number of days. I was tempted to say "several" days, but these days, they try to get you out of the hospital as quickly as possible. As one doctor said to me, "People get sick in hospitals!" That wasn't very reassuring when I first heard the statement, but it's absolutely true!

When you first get into your hospital bed, a feeling of calm may come over you. The thought that you might even get comfortable starts to form in your mind. *This bed isn't that bad. At least my room has a window. Boy, those nurses sure are nice.* Thoughts of this nature are common at the very beginning. You start to play with the buttons on the bed — up and down, tilt, raise the legs, lower the head — and then there is the television. Usually, they never spend a lot on satellite or cable service. Why should they? It's assumed that you are either sick or recovering from some major surgery. If it were minor surgery, you wouldn't be in the hospital to begin with. Your designation would be the coveted "outpatient" category. If that is the case, then you can skip this entire chapter, unless your "outpatient" procedure goes South. Then you will need some of the information that I am applying here.

Once you are situated in your room (hopefully, it is a private room to start with), there are a few things to know. Do not allow anyone to move your end table far out of your reach. Make sure that the nurse doesn't leave until you check to see that everything necessary is close at hand. Ask for a pitcher of ice water. This may sound elementary, my dear Watson, but it happens: Everyone leaves, and there isn't any water on your "table" — the rolling table they push over your legs. Sometimes these are the fancy kind with a drawer and fancy flip-up thing with a mirror. It's always nice to see what kind of a wreck you look like. Most of the time, these are the cheaper variety, with a simple, flat surface, a device that allows the entire table to slide up and down, and, of course, the wheels. Remember what I told you before: *Everything* in a hospital *always* has a set of wheels.

One thing to watch out for is this: A nurse will come into your room and go about the standard checks. Then they pull out the covers down by your feet; they always have to feel your feet, for some reason. The problem is, they never put the covers back, and you are left with exposed toes! The worst part is that you're not able to correct this oversight. A person in your condition will not be able to reach the foot of the bed, especially when you have a bunch of staples holding your internal organs together. Make sure they replace your covers. Yes, the nurse will probably make a face because they hate to make your bed. It is the orderlies' or housekeeping's job to do that. But, if you don't insist, you'll be living with cold feet for a number of hours.

At first there will be a bunch of wires and monitors attached to you. One will be the oxygen sensor, which is always on the end of one of your fingers. The little red light measures the amount of oxygen in your hemoglobin. That's all I know about that thing, so please don't ask. It has always been a mystery to me how it works — a little red light shining on your fingernail tells you how much oxygen is in your blood! The only problem with having the device on your finger is trying to eat! But hold on a minute, pilgrim — I forgot one important point: If you just came up from surgery, they won't *give* you anything to eat. You will be on a clear-liquid diet, and this will consist of broth, more broth, and a little more broth. There won't even be a saltine on your tray. The doctor will decide how long you stay on the clear-liquid diet. On the bright side, look at how much weight you will be losing. There might be sherbet on the tray; Italian Ice is considered to be clear liquid. If there isn't, ask, and I will tell you why.

Every floor has access to a refrigerator/freezer and a cabinet full of goodies. They keep all kinds of snacks behind closed doors, and the freezer is stocked with little cups of ice cream that even have a spoon attached to the lid of the container. I don't know who did this first, the airlines or the hospitals, but it is always there. Usually all you have to do is ask. But don't get greedy. If you're on a clear-liquid diet, don't ask for ice cream — that isn't a clear liquid. Ask for the sherbet, or Italian ice, and do not quibble about the flavor — not at this stage of your hospital stay. Whatever flavor they give you will taste really good. That's the thing about being in the hospital — it is called *deprivation*. If a family member brings in a pocket full of Snicker bars, don't eat them if you are on a clear-liquid diet. Don't eat anything you can't see through. There is a very good reason for this. If they have to run you back into the OR for some reason, they don't want to find a stomach full of nougat or peanuts

The Chronicles of Pain

floating around in there. It will definitely ruin both your doctor's day and your own.

After you are given a solid-food diet, try not to hoard things. If there is cantaloupe on your tray and you're not going to eat it, don't stash it in your end table for later. Just send it back. After a few days, you will have a drawer full of sugar packets, applesauce cups, a few extra Salisbury steaks, and probably a nest of rodents. You don't have to stash food everywhere, nor do you have to save it for your relatives — they won't want your hospital condiments. Simply do not order it, or just leave the stuff on your tray — someone will sneak in and make it go away. Keep in mind the pantry down the hall, stocked full of tasty tidbits. They will even have Oreo cookies and Lorna Doones. When was the last time you saw a package of Lorna Doones? And, there will be ice cream.

If your husband brings in a thermos of iced tea every day and it smells a little bit like almonds, he is trying to whack you for the insurance money. It's got arsenic in it, and it will kill you. Of course, some of the food the hospital sends up from the kitchens will look pretty suspicious, also. I have seen things that do not exist outside of the hospital-kitchen environment: Strange-looking vegetables and fish sticks, weird little things that you would normally use on Halloween to scare the kiddies with. Hopefully, that won't happen to you. There is a hospital in Boca Raton, Florida, where you can order a bottle of Rothschild 1939 Bordeaux. This was the same facility that the neurosurgeon who fixed my back operated out of — the guy with the $500K Italian sports car. If no one has ever told you, the really big money is not in Palm Beach — it's in Gulf Stream and Boca Raton. As far as these people are concerned, only peons live in Palm Beach!

It almost goes without saying that life can be boring when you are lying in a hospital bed for any length of time. For that reason, small things become very important — that cup of coffee on your morning tray, the small cup of Jello in the afternoon, and a dinner feast of all edible things.

Before we go any further, let's take a moment to look at *visiting hours*.

Years ago, they used to be very strict about visiting hours, usually 7:00 p.m. to 9:00 p.m. — no exceptions! In today's recovery experience, that has changed. It seems like visitors can show up at practically any time, day or night. For some of my final surgeries, I used to prefer to have no visitors at all. When I would fly up to Scranton from Charleston, I would tell my wife to just stay home and that I would see her in a week or so. This isn't cruel — there is actually solid logic behind this approach, and I'll explain why. Being in a hospital bed for several days is like going to war. It's best not to have a wife, girlfriend, or boyfriend, for that matter, somewhere in the United States while you're traipsing around a jungle with a bazooka. There is nothing to distract you, no "Dear John" letters to upset you, especially at the wrong moment. I know this because my Uncle Sam provided me with the opportunity to carry out his orders in a Southeast Asian "resort."

Look at it this way: You find out that there will be a really good movie on television at 8:00 p.m. You look forward to that all day — that and your daily allotment of Jello. Just when the movie is about to come on, Aunt Melba and Uncle Toast show up. It's 7:45, and you are pissed because you know that they aren't going to leave in 15 minutes. So, you keep the movie on but turn the volume off; you try to watch it while still making eye contact with them.

It won't take long for the question to be asked. It is the universal hospital-bed inquiry, the question you dread hearing, and it usually goes like this: "How are you doing?" *Well, considering my circumstances, I should think that the answer is rather obvious: I'm lying here in a hospital bed with tubes coming out of every orifice of my body, but other than that, I am feeling just stupendous. And I will tell you something else: If you help me out of this bed, I will do the limbo right here on the floor. I would prefer to go horseback riding, but that may require a gown with the back portion intact.*

Another bane of a hospital patient. The visitors who come at dinnertime. Believe me, their timing is not always coincidental — after a few days, you might detect a pattern. The orderly brings your tray in with a cheery hello: "Hello Mr. Bandages. I have some nice provisions for you. Oh! I see you have a guest. Well, I'll just pop this right here and be on my way." This is the cue for your guest to ask the first question: "How is the food here?" You answer that it isn't bad until you learn to dodge the question, or you say, "It's not fit for humans." The guest will then offer to cut up your meat and vegetables for you; it is at this point where a piece of your long-awaited pork chop goes into his or her mouth. They will wave this off by saying it was a test to see if it was hot enough for you. If, for any reason, you stumble with the cutlery, your dinner is history, because the guest will offer to feed you, and your ego will just not allow that to happen. In fact, you would rather starve to death before allowing someone to do that for you, so you say, "Ah, the hell with it. You go ahead and eat that gruel. I wasn't that hungry anyway. They

The Chronicles of Pain

gave me a big lunch!"

Then you will get the specialized food vultures, the ones who can see a nice dessert from a mile away. These are the culprits who go only for the good stuff — Jello or a piece of sheet cake with buttercream icing — the desserts you live for when locked away in a hospital bed. You'll gobble up part of everything on the tray just to get to that ultimate prize — cake, pudding, or two sugar cookies. It will infuriate you that this person is trying to get first dibs on your treasured dessert. But it's your wife's sister — what in the hell are you supposed to say? "Hey, get the fuck away from that cake! If you even *think* of eating my Jello, there *will* be consequences."

These are a few of the pitfalls of being confined to a hospital bed. But it can always get worse. During the day, you might find yourself dozing off. There is a reason for that. Every night, as soon as you fall asleep, someone will come in with the biggest needle you've ever seen and tell you to turn the other cheek. Yep, it hurts like hell because it feels like they are injecting battery acid into your ass. After the pain subsides enough for you to fall asleep again — bingo! They wake you up again to do "vitals." Keep in mind that the shift will change, and, every time that happens, a new batch of nurses will converge on your territory.

They will proceed to check your "vitals" again, or the drug lady will have a little paper cup full of pills for you to swallow while they watch. Don't ever ask them what a certain pill is for. Once you do that, the word will get around the control desk that you are "particular." They will start referring to you as *Doctor Patient in 304*, the person who has memorized the *PDR*.

Do you know what that is? *PDR* stands for: ***P**hysicians **D**esk **R**eference*. This is a huge book — about 18,000 pages — that contains every drug known to man, dating back to the Paleolithic period. It has color glossy photos of all of the common narcotic medications and print so small that you need an electron microscope to read it. This book is on every doctor's desk somewhere. Actually, I take that back: The *PDR* requires its own purpose-built desk to keep it on, or the entire thing will crash down through the floor. An interesting side note: Back in the hippy-dippy days (I am referring to the 1960s and 1970s — you know, back before dirt was invented), this was the Bible of your neighborhood commune drug dealer. It would tell a person with a fifth-grade education which pills would get you high and which ones would cause diarrhea. Sort of like that Jefferson Airplane song, "White Rabbit": *"The one that Mother gives you/won't do anything at all/Go ask Alice/When you're ten feet tall...."*

The Chronicles of Pain

The big day has arrived. They have been instructed to remove your catheter — you'll be free from the tube! But I wouldn't count your gauze pads just yet — there is more to come, a lot more.

The night before one of my major back surgeries, I had my wife track down a hairstylist to give me a trim prior to the big event. The gentleman who showed up was quite amiable, but he did exhibit a few feminine qualities often encountered in his profession. My surgeon at the time was going through his mid-life crazy period. He divorced his wife for a 20-something-year-old, went out and bought a Porsche, and started to dress like the population of Monaco. He came into my room and saw this entire menagerie taking place, and his facial expression changed immediately. It was even more apparent once my hairstylist said, "Well, *hello*, Doctor, it's so nice to see you…" Well, he just flipped out, turned on his heel, and stormed out. You must understand that he was a "manly man," and this introduction just didn't cut it.

The next morning, while I was being prepped for surgery, he asked me what that demonstration was all about, and I explained to him what I'm about to tell you. Get your hair cut *before* you have a major surgical intervention. The reason is simple: You won't see the inside of a shower stall for a week. Plus, that "dry shampoo" they give you is garbage. It's a powder that you rub into your hair and then brush it out. *Voila!* Your hair will still feel greasy. I don't know about you, but I hate that feeling, having a greasy head of hair. Of course, if you are bald, just ignore this last paragraph.

Another thing that you must know about are the coveted *Nurse Call* buttons. As soon as you are situated in your new home, someone will show you the nurse call button. They will tell you that, if you need anything, just push that button, and someone will come running. That, of course, is under laboratory conditions; in the real world, different responses will apply. For example, if you hit that button when the nurses are changing shift — good luck. It will depend on what button you push. If you use the one in the bathroom — assuming that you can *get* to the bathroom — they will be there Johnny on the Spot. The only problem with that is, unless you are lying on the bathroom floor with various parts of your intestines falling out, they will be really pissed off at you for using *that* button. Here is what I did once in 1983 after one of my back surgeries.

In the old days, they used to attach you to the rack and start asking you questions about your trip to Moscow. But nowadays, they want you to get out of bed as quickly as possible after your procedure, and they want you to walk as much as possible. At first, your walking will be monitored by a nurse. Then as time rolls by, they will provide you with a "walker," one of those tubular aluminum deals that immediately age you 50 years. And finally, you will be given a smiley face button and a cane with six legs sticking out of the bottom.

One day I was doing my walking laps around the 8th floor with my multi-legged cane when I spied an open door. Lo and behold, inside was a human skeleton hanging from one of those wheeled bases. Remember the second idiom: *Everything has wheels*, including the toilet bowl. Anyway, I threw a sheet over my bony accomplice and rolled him/her into my room. Then I quickly transferred my friend to my bed, pulled up the covers, and then — the *pièce de résistance* — I placed the nurse call button in its bony little hand. I pushed the button and ran and hid in the bathroom. Naturally, there was a big scream. It turned out that this nurse was new to the floor. A bunch of backup nurses came running in, and there was extreme chaos.

That night, my surgeon, the same one who had dealt so well with my alternative-lifestyle hairdresser, came into my room. The first thing he said was, "Jason, what the hell are you doing to my nurses?" In typical 1960s protest anything mode, I said, "Doctor, that was a protest. I was making a statement as to how long it takes to get a pain shot around here!" He wasn't impressed and chewed me out some more, telling me never to do that again, blah, blah, blah. Secretly, though, I think he liked it because he knew my history as an artist and writer. This doctor introduced me to Jason Miller, the guy who wrote some pretty big plays and starred in the first *Exorcist* movie as the young priest who got tossed down the stone steps. Not that this information has much to do with what we were discussing.

My point is simple. When you first arrive on the "floor," you will be treated like royalty, but as your condition improves, the little nurse call button will not necessarily have them running at your beck and call. It pays to try to figure out when they change shifts. That way, you can get in your request before they talk about what a pain in the ass you are, and you can start raiding the snack cabinet.

"Jello" is a brand name. I guess there should be an asterisk beside it, but my lawyer will let me know if it is needed. In the hospital they give this particular food product fancy names like "Gelatin Jewels" or "Belly Dancer Delight" — anything but "Jello." That would assume they are serving you the real thing — you know, the one without the rubber on top. This is a prime dessert on any hospital tray, but there is one situation that could doom your entire culinary adventure while a guest of a hospital. It's called "The Low Sodium Diet." What is even worse is the infamous "Low Fat Diet." If that happens, you are truly screwed. *Low salt*, you might be able to live with, but, *low fat* — that is a different story entirely. What "low fat" means is this: No taste, plain and simple, *nada*, nope, *nyet*, forget taste. I have been on low-fat diets on a number of occasions, and it is a fate worse than — well, I can't say "death" — it just *sucks*! Excuse my use of the "King's English," but I can't think of another word right now to explain the ramifications of a low-fat diet.

A person does not realize how tasteless food is without any fat content. It's true: No fat, no taste. One day the orderly came in with my tray, and, with great flourish, he whipped the cover off of the plate. Sitting there was *one* piece of fish, about 2 inch square and 1 inch thick. Next to the fish, which had a slice of lemon on it for effect, were eight — I counted them — eight green beans. I don't mean *entire* green beans. These were pieces, cut Julienne style, without butter or salt. And, to wrap up this sumptuous banquet of earthly delights, there was one-quarter cup of wild rice. I knew that for a fact because the paperwork came with the meal. And to top it all off was a half-cup of sugar-free gelatin jewels. That was my dinner for the entire evening. The secret hall cabinet I told you about, the one stocked full of Oreos, Lorna Doones, and ice cream in a variety of flavors, was deemed off limits to me.

Now let me tell you what happens at mealtime in a hospital. The entire corridor fills with the smell of food. It is a universal scent, not individual aromas but a combination of everything rolled into one sensory appeal. In comparison, my dinner didn't have any smell at all — even the fish was without scent. Oh, I take that back: The lemon slice *did* smell like lemon, which I suppose it was required by law to smell like. I lay in that bed, just being bombarded by this sensory overload. My sense of smell was expediently more acute due to the number of days I was on this low-sodium, no-fat diet. I could transport myself right into that Irish potato the guy in the next room was eating. My body was screaming for salt, fat, taste — *anything.* I would even consider a tempura dog dropping if the presentation was done correctly. A little ginger on the side and a small pile of wasabi tastefully placed near the dog turd. I can see it as clear as day, my Sushi chef, with the black-and-white bandana wrapped around his head, bowing to me and saying, in a very low voice; "Dog roll, *anjisan!*" (a reference from *Shogun.*)

I'm not known for my "Helpful Hints" column in the local newspaper, because it doesn't exist.

The Chronicles of Pain

But I will toss one your way free of charge. If you arrive at the floor where your patient is located and have forgotten a little gift or a get-well card, don't panic. Look for a plastic glove dispenser; they are usually hanging on the wall somewhere, and it *will* be there with this virus going around. Find yourself a glove, if you have to, and take it into the restroom to do this. Place a folded paper towel down and use it as a cushion. Take out your ballpoint pen and very gently write, "Get Well," and then sign it. Now, blow the thing up until it looks like a cow's udder with all of the *tea-ats* hanging down. Well, yours will be sticking out in different angles. There is a reason for that — the cow is just full of milk.

That's it! This is your get-well card. After everyone makes a big fuss over it, carefully pin it to the corkboard. You will be the hit of the floor. People will come up from the boiler room just to see your innovative get-well message. Have some tissues handy, because there will be tears shed, profusely, over your massively thoughtful gift.

Wardrobe: Do not bring your Gucci purse to the hospital. Don't wear anything that has sequins on it. They are going to take away your clothing at their first opportunity and put it in a plastic bag with your name and VIN number. In today's age, there will be a handful of self-stick labels with a barcode on them. They will stick these things everywhere they can. After you go home, there will be a barcode stuck to your forehead. Usually that bag of clothes will be stuffed under your rolling bed. Or, they may put rollers on it so that they can roll it around with you like an appendage.

If, for any reason, you wake up dressed in hospital scrubs, hide them. Don't tell anyone that you have a set of scrubs. If you do, lose them — it's that simple. There is a reason I'm telling you this, like there is for everything else in this book. I know because I have experienced everything that I'm talking about 45 times.[3]

Hospital scrubs are some of the most comfortable clothing in the entire world. This is especially true if they have been washed a billion times. If you are fortunate enough to be dressed in a set of scrubs prior to being placed in your room, then consider it *manna* from the hospital *stupa*. Fold these things up, and hide them in your own, personal clothing bag with the UPC code emblazoned on the side. Any two-piece ensemble will serve you faithfully as

---

[3]That isn't a typo. I have had 45 major surgical interventions or extreme near-death experiences in the hospital. The most recent involved the COVID-19 virus. I was infected with that on May 13, 2020. But that story is in the next chapter. If you want to cheat and jump ahead, go on and do it. If it helps you maintain social distance and wear a mask, then my task is completed.

The Chronicles of Pain

loungewear for many years to come, and you won't have to marry a doctor to get a set, unless your internal organs prove to be love at first sight. That's different.

Another thing about hospital rooms to remember is this: *Don't walk around barefoot.* The people at the nursing station are nuts about people falling. They will chew you a new one if they catch you walking around in your bare feet. You must always put on those ridiculous "Moon shoes." That's what I call those things with the bumps all over the bottom. As gross as your moon shoes may seem, always wear them. Never, ever wear them in bed. The sheets will stick to the bottoms, and you will have your feet near your head all night. Always remove them before you go to bed. Speaking of gross, I'm not sure I would trust walking around barefoot anywhere in a hospital, especially my own room. One thing that you will notice is that nurses drop things a lot. More importantly, the object in question stays dropped until housekeeping eventually comes and sweeps the joint.

There will be all kinds of things on the floor in your room after a few days. There will be plastic devices under your bed, along with the homeless person who moved in while you were in surgery. Bits of paper, probably enough to build a campfire, will be down there.

Those plastic caps that protect the needles? Yep, they'll be there, too, if you look hard enough. The floor in your room will become a virtual junkyard of medical waste products. Sometimes you can request housekeeping to come up and "do" your room, but you have to go through Nurse Diesel with that request. If you are the pain-in-the-ass-patient-in-room-408, your request may have an accident getting to the proper individuals. Diesel will tell you that your request committed suicide right after she sent it — something about a lost inheritance or a love affair that went South. If that happens, just start throwing your food on the floor and against the walls — that is sure to get their attention. It may also get you a straitjacket for a few days.

Perfumes and Aftershave: Please leave these at home. If you come in for surgery and reek of English Leather, they won't touch you with a knife. They will send you home because your pre-op instructions will have said *Do Not* wear perfume or aftershave. As with everything else in this epistle, there is a reason for this request. Some people are allergic to heavy scents; others find them very distracting while operating. You would be better off with a non-distracted surgeon when he is cutting you open with an electric saw. Your hospital room is a very expensive rental property while you are a guest of any given hospital. They would prefer if you did not rearrange the furniture or douse everything with Chanel Number Five. That is not recommended; it's not a good idea on any day. The best you will be able to do is arrange all of the cow-udder get-well cards on your cork board. Or stack up your meager number of clothes nice and neat in your wardrobe — but that's about it. It is a temporary environment — at least we hope that is the case!

You can walk into a hospital bare naked, and all of your basic needs will be met. They will supply wearing apparel. It may not enhance the color of your eyes, but it will suffice at covering your body. Unless you happen to stumble into a "clothing optional" facility, in that case, a Rolex and a big smile should see you through. The toiletries may all have strange-sounding brand names, but they will pretty much do the jobs they're intended for. I really can't address the issue of leg and underarm shaving, but I can definitely relate.

There are other issues that are unique to hospitals that we should address. One of them is the drawing of blood, also known as "phlebotomy." I sometimes refer to phlebotomists as "vampires," which is very nice until you find two punctures in your neck after they leave.

Not all phlebotomists are created or trained

equally. I have had some who have to stick me several times until I threaten them with role reversal. Actually, in today's hospitals, I think they can't poke you more than two or three times. Any number above that, they have to call in "Vlad the Impaler." She is the nurse who has been there since they invented the concept of blood. Vlad rarely ever misses the mark.

Years ago, I spent 21 days in "French Hospital," San Francisco. Because of the particular disorder I was suffering from, they had to draw blood every morning. At 6:00 a.m. sharp, the same guy came into my room with his little tray of vials. This man was of Japanese descent; he would come in and bow — not a word was ever spoken. He would then get his needle ready and place it on my arm. Then, with a loud "*Hai!*" in went the needle exactly, every time. The guy would then bow again, and quietly leave, closing the door behind himself. A lot of nurses and technicians never close the door; doctors are notorious for always leaving the door open when they depart unless you tell them otherwise. This is important to remember; you can't just jump out of bed and close a door.

Blood, doors, lights — what has this got to do with a hospital stay? The short answer is *everything*. By the time you get into a hospital bed, it's a given that you haven't been knitting quilts lately. Something is radically wrong with your body; it has malfunctioned, and a bunch of high-priced specialists are trying to correct the disorder. The point is to have as much quality of life while you are confined to a hospital bed as possible. That is the goal of this book: I am trying to provide you with a few well-learned mistakes to avoid and make your stay as beneficial as possible as you while away the hours. Speaking of which, here is another true story centered around one of my hospital experiences after having a major surgery.

I am going to have to give you a brief history prior to relating this next story. Back in the mid-1980s, a friend of mine who was in the automobile business, quite successful, I might add, became involved with some seedy "partners" in a construction venture. My pal was supposed to be nothing but a "silent partner," which means that he put up a pile of money. Well, the entire thing went to hell, and Charles called me one day, begging me to take the reins of this construction business as the general manager. I spent about a week looking at all of the books and various records and told my friend that all I could do was simply lessen the blow of his loss. In other words, I would be able to break even on these government contracts and stem the flow of his additional capital going into this sinking ship. One of the jobs that I inherited involved rebuilding a fire station in a town outside of Scranton, Pennsylvania. I won't name the place, and you will understand why in a few minutes.

I hired a crew of competent people and went about the task of completing these contracts, with one being the fire station in blah, blah, Pennsylvania. There were bribes to be paid and a few other under-the-table deals made in order to bring this job in under budget and on time. When you work in Northeastern Pennsylvania, you find out quickly that it is like a third-world country when it comes to getting anything done without greasing a number of palms — and I don't mean the trees. So, I greased away, and the job was done. My buddy came out not losing as much money as he thought he was going to, and I packed up my car and left for Florida, because the snow was getting ready to fly in the Wilkes-Barre/Scranton area.

Years passed, and I was in the CMC hospital, having another back surgery, when one evening, while on one of my walks around the corridors, I strolled past the lounge and I heard a voice say, "Hey, buddy — I know youse, don't I?" I looked and recognized him as one of the "officials" that I had to deal with on the fire-station project. Naturally, his name was "Tony," and, yes, I remembered him.

There was my good old buddy Tony, sitting in the lounge, and surrounded by three big guys wearing black leather sport coats. Tony waved to me. "Hey, goomba, com' ear, com' ear — let me introduce youse to my boys." Tony was sitting there, holding court, wearing his elaborate silk bathrobe and $500 slippers. He patted the cushion next to him and told me to sit down. "Yo, Goodman — that's it, ain't it? Goodman, these are my main guys, Crusher, Low Blow, and that bum o'er dere, we call Itchy Knuckles. Say hello to my good friend Goodman, boys." They all got up, one at a time, and shook my hand. While they were doing so, I noticed the unmistakable shape of a 9mm handgun under their jackets. As fate would have it, my Goomba buddy was in there for some follow-up surgery on his heart, but this didn't affect his appetite or his thirst. They were eating Italian cheese, salami, and some stuffed shells, washing it down with a bottle of Dago Red. After the little snack, out came the bottle of Crown Royal, and we proceeded to sit there getting sloshed in the lounge on the 8th floor of the CMC hospital in Scranton, Pennsylvania. Tony went on to say, "Youse listen to me, Tony. Goodman — anythin' youse need, just ask. If anybody gives youse a hard time, just tell me, Tony, an' I'll have it fixed." Do you know what? Tony wasn't joking. He'd made a lot of money off of that firehouse project, and this was his way of saying "Thanks."

This nightly event went on for about three more days. Every night, his boys would come in with this huge sack full of the evening's offerings: good Italian food, wine, and top-shelf liquor. Tony owned a strip club in the "No Name" town. He even asked me if I needed some "company" for the night! I'm sure that, had I said "Yes," some girl named Penny Nickels would have shown up at my room, and it wouldn't have been to change my bandages. I can tell you this: That was the safest I ever felt after having a back surgery — not to mention the introduction of an alternative to hospital food and beverages!

The Chronicles of Pain

Chapter Four

Days and Nights with the Coronavirus

The Chronicles of Pain

The COVID-19 virus pandemic isn't slowing down. In fact, it's getting worse. Hopefully, something that I say over the next handful of pages may have some effect on someone out there and persuade them to at least wear a mask. The story you are about to read is true and factual to the best of my knowledge. You must understand — there is a lot of confusion associated with this COVID-19 virus infection. It has taken me months to sit here in front of this typewriter and put two sentences together that make sense. I am sure there are a few out there who may beg to differ on that statement, but it's true. I have come into my studio several times over the last few months, sat down in front of this typewriter, and just stared. If this is called "writer's block," then mine was a case of "writer's blockhouse."

I sketched the outline and basic format of this book a few years ago, and over that period of time, I would add a few pages of notes when something flashed into my mind about my many hospital stays. But I can tell you this with all sincerity: This last hospital encounter — a lengthy stay, in a coma, with the COVID-19 virus — I would not wish on my mortal enemy. This virus is nothing to take lightly. In the following pages, I may make a crack or two, or even produce a play on words that may elicit a bit of laughter. But rest assured — there is nothing funny or humorous about having this virus and fighting for one's life. You, as the reader, almost didn't have *The Chronicles of Pain* on your nightstand — it was that close. So please accept my apologies, if any are needed, for making the next chapter about a virus that is killing Americans.

The following story about AA meetings and recovery houses may seem like a digression for a chapter that is supposed to be about my experience with the COVID-19 virus. But please: Indulge me while I set the stage for a very grim episode in my life.

May 13, 2020 was the day my friend Doug asked me if I wanted to attend a barbecue and meeting in some small town near Ephrata, Pennsylvania. I agreed to this, because they closed not only the liquor stores in Pennsylvania but also, in their infinite wisdom, all of the AA meetings, too! Normally, I am quite guarded about my involvement with Alcoholics Anonymous. I have been sober for more than 34 years at the time of this writing. But there is a saying in AA: "You can't keep it if you don't give it away...." I guess you could say that I was eager to give something away that day. Most of the meetings had shut down in February. By the middle of May 2020, it became abundantly clear that this virus was nothing to trifle with.

It was around this time that people started to die *en masse*, and our leaders in Washington seemed to be doing everything in their power to make sure that trend continued.

So, Doug came to my house; we piled into my Mustang GT and made our way to this "event." When we arrived, the host was in the kitchen, preparing something for that night's offering. The deal was this: John, the host, had a deck on the back of his house with a gas-fired grill. He would cook up a batch of hot dogs, or in this case, German sausages, people would bring other food items, and they would cobble together a meal. After dinner, everyone would retire to the barn in the backyard, and they would hold an AA meeting.

When Doug and I arrived, there wasn't anyone else there besides John. We sat on stools in the kitchen area and made small talk while John prepared whatever he was working on at the kitchen sink. After about 45 minutes, the front door flew open, and in poured about 25 guys, all in their early 30s. It turns out that these people were all clients at various recovery houses around the area, and that is who John was entertaining each week.

If you are not familiar with the recovery-house concept, allow me to explain it. Individuals set up these residences and sometimes get paid by the state to house these recovering alcohol and drug addicts. They are segregated by sex, so there are both male and female houses. Usually, when someone leaves a 30-day treatment program, they go on to a longer stay in one of these recovery houses. Sometimes it can be up to one or two years, though most of them are in the six-month range. There are rules in these places: You cannot use the drug of your choice; if that behavior is detected, they will throw you out onto the street.

After a month or so, you are required to get a "sponsor." I mentioned this earlier and, at the time, declined to explain the process, but, here, I will go into a little depth defining it. This is an AA and NA concept; "sponsor" doesn't mean that the person has to contact Coca-Cola or the Ford Motor Company and ask for financial backing. A "sponsor" is a person with some longer-term sobriety who helps a new person get acclimated to the 12-step program. You could say that a sponsor is a *guide* who shows the newcomer how to navigate life without the use of chemicals or booze. The recovery-house concept requires the resident to get a job after a month or two. Now, keep in mind, none of this stuff is free. Somehow, someone is paying the tab — usually the welfare office or the Medicaid program. I had a guy tell me once that he'd been in 15 recovery treatment programs. My response was to explain to him that the U.S. Navy trains jet pilots for less than that was costing the taxpayers. Needless to say, our relationship grew sour rather quickly after that.

I have attended AA all over the world. One in particular comes to mind. My wife and I were spending several days in Amsterdam. As we walked around the city, we passed numerous hashish and pot bars. You could order from a menu of various style "hash" or marijuana products, and they would bring it to your table. They usually served fruit juice or coffee with your order. Rarely did they have alcoholic beverages at these places. Anyway, after seeing this all over the city, I went to an English-language AA meeting at a local hospital. After the meeting, in conversation with one of the counselors who worked there, it turns out that a resident is allowed only *one* treatment experience at the taxpayers' expense. After that, if you still needed treatment, *you* had to pony up all of the cash for any future treatment. I found that quite interesting and hence the comment to our future jet-fighter pilot.

Now, where was I? Oh, yes — the recovery house. One thing that I learned that evening was the fact that a number of 30-year-old gentlemen have made the recovery house their career choice. As it was explained, they go out and get all messed up on meth, and when the situation becomes untenable, they go into a treatment program somewhere, and then back to a recovery house. I would imagine that it would beat the rigors of a Wall Street career any day.

So, in essence, that is where I was infected with the coronavirus — at an AA meeting, trying to do the right thing.

Prior to May 13, 2020, things were somewhat bleak here in central Pennsylvania, with this outbreak changing people's lives overnight. It reminded me of Gabriel García Marquez and his depiction of life in *Love in the Time of Cholera*.... We weren't going anywhere or doing anything that we were supposed to be doing. In mid-March, Teresa and I were booked on flights to Ireland. We had to be there before the first of April to renegotiate the lease on our apartment. Naturally, that trip was canceled, as well as all subsequent trips, like going to Puerto Vallarta to use our timeshare at the Melia resort. (If you're interested in owning a timeshare with the Melia group, let me know. I have one for sale *all* the time!)

Instead of going to Ireland, we decided to work on our house. The garage doors needed to be stripped and painted, as did a portion of the brick on our house. So, we hunkered down and

The Chronicles of Pain

worked on the house. Our house is an old (ca. 1908) "robber baron" mansion of sorts in a small and rather popular Amish town. A few years ago, our town was voted the "Coolest Town in America" by some big travel magazine. This was the kiss of death for our quiet lifestyle. The exact thing happened in Ireland — the little village we live in there was voted the "Best Place in Ireland to Live," and that ruined that place. As soon as tourists found out that they could buy a house here — and there — they came in droves. Now, Lititz, Pennsylvania, is full of "Over 55" living arrangements — and recovery houses, of course.

We were working away, starting at the middle of April, as soon as the weather broke. (I've never understood the term *the weather broke*. What does it mean? A big crack forms in the sky?) We painted, scraped, and painted some more, and then went on to do some garden work. I ordered a couple yards of mulch and had it delivered. We had just started to spread the mulch around the yard when we both seemed to run out of energy real fast. It had gotten so bad that I could barely push a wheelbarrow load — despite the fact that our backyard is almost flat. Plus, if you've ever spread mulch, you know that it doesn't have very much weight to it at all.

That reminds me of something else. Mulch!

Every year my neighbor, the architect, goes out and hauls in loads of mulch in his huge Dodge Ram pickup truck. It seems like an exercise in futility: You spend all that money, work like a dog to spread the stuff, and then it just disappears over the course of the summer, or someone comes in at night and steals it. After being discharged from the hospital — and when I could walk and talk at the same time — we decided to take on another project in the front yard. I had my Mennonite contractor come in and replace the front porch. The money I saved by not going to Ireland was put to good use on that project. We used all man-made materials so that I never have to scrape and paint — or have someone else do it at great expense. Even the decking is a composite, guaranteed to last into the next century. My contractor and his sons poured a new sidewalk for us, and we decided to re-landscape the front yard. But this time, I went to Home Depot and bought bags of rubber mulch. Yep, that's correct — it's made of ground-up tires and comes in both black and brown. The stuff is also guaranteed to last until the pyramids collapse — and it was about the same price as the regular mulch. The most expensive part of the job was a digital camera surveillance system I had installed to catch the culprits who were stealing my backyard mulch.

Working in the backyard gave me my first

indication that something was wrong. I was always extremely tired, and I found myself getting confused a lot. Some people would say that happens when you turn 70, but this was something else. I would take naps in the middle of the day. I am not accustomed to taking naps. It wasn't something my German workaholic father would allow me to do during the day when he was paying me to operate a bulldozer. Plus, my sense of taste and smell just faded into oblivion. Now, that *could* have been the result of my cooking, but it was a little hard to believe. When you can't tase a load of garlic, something is definitely wrong. Then, on the holiday weekend, Memorial Day weekend, the poop really hit the fan. I was fucked! I have no recall from about May 23 onward. It's a complete blank, like a blackout from drinking too much, gone forever.

On May 23, 2020, Teresa drove me to the Veterans Medical Center in Lebanon, Pennsylvania. The drive is 18.6 miles one way, and I have made this trip on numerous occasions because this is my "go to" place for all of my services connected to disabilities. She told me afterward that I didn't say anything except for one incident. Teresa was driving my Mustang GT convertible. It has the "Shaker 500" sound system — this thing actually has speakers in the seats! She dialed in a Patsy Cline album.

She said that I just turned to her and said, "Pig Squeezens," which is a rather derogatory comment on country-western music. She said it was the only thing that I said for the entire trip. Teresa told me that she knew right then that I hadn't lost my sense of humor!

At the Emergency Room, they came out with a wheelchair and loaded me into it. The staff would not allow Teresa to come into the hospital. Just think — that was the last time we saw each other until June 22, when I was discharged — 30 days later!

They checked my oxygen levels with that little device that they place on one of your fingers. It has the red light in it and somehow figures out how much oxygen you have in your blood. Amazing! When they checked me that morning, my "O" level was 30 percent!!! Do you realize what that means? I was almost dead. Doctors have given that condition a name — they call it "Happy Hypoxia." It is a characteristic of the COVID-19 virus that is not fully understood. The medical people are amazed that a patient can converse and appear "normal" and yet have an "O" level that would normally be attributed to a dead man.

After receiving that meter reading, the leading physician in the ER went outside and asked Teresa for permission to put me on a ventilator. This was the first of her agonies;

The Chronicles of Pain

many more would follow as this portrait was painted. In hindsight, I can tell you this: There was nothing "happy" about it for Teresa! She actually suffered more than I did during this early stage of the infection.

I don't know if you're familiar with this whole ventilator thing or not. But allow me to explain the basics. The ventilator is so uncomfortable, they have to put you into a coma. This is normally done with drugs. But one of the drawbacks to a ventilator is that your body gets a vacation from making you breathe. This is problematic, because, after a period of time, your own body will refuse to go back to work, and that is a very serious condition. I remember vaguely when they brought me out of the coma to check my ability to breathe on my own. As one doctor explained to me, they bring you out of this chemically induced coma to check that you are still alive.

Later that day, I was transported (or so I'm told) from the Veterans Medical Center to a civilian hospital called LGH — Lancaster General Hospital. Now you must remember one important thing here: From this point on, my memory is more than a little fuzzy on the details about my stay at LGH. I remember almost nothing from May 23 until a few days before discharge, just shy of June 22, 2020. It would be easy to attribute my sketchy memory to age, but I am convinced that this COVID-19 thing has affected it, also. I'd be in the middle of a conversation with someone, and, in the middle of a sentence, my mind would just draw a complete blank. I could almost see the word that I wanted to say, but I couldn't put it into its place. This has been happening a lot since my battle against the COVID-19 infection.

I was told that, at LGH, I was in a serious state of confusion. They asked me what year it was, and I had no idea. Then I was asked what my name was, and guess what? I had not a clue as to who I was.

At one point, they called Teresa and asked her if I was a violent person. She responded, "No" and asked why they were asking that. A doctor went on to say that I had ripped out my ventilator tube and all of the wires attached to my chest. I don't remember any of this, but I will say this: After this incident, my hands were tied to the bedrails with nylon straps. I recall thinking that I was being held in some kind of experimental facility or prison. I asked the nurse for some paper, but I couldn't write. My hands and fingers simply refused to cooperate! They handed me a small plastic thing that looked like a device from Babylon. My secret message would be punched out on a clay tablet with a wedge-shaped spoon stylus.

When I tried to write, I could not make any

The Chronicles of Pain

letters — it was just a series of scribbles. Then the nurse would say, in that *nurse* type of way, "Maybe *we'll* try this tomorrow; does that sound good?" *Not exactly, my dear.* At this point in time, I felt like I was in one of Warren Zevon's songs — *"Send lawyers, guns and money/How was I to know/she was with the Russians, too?"* Sure, I'm making light of a serious situation, but that's the point. How else am I supposed to process this without some humor? Being in a weird place, totally unfamiliar territory, with people walking around in those "Hazmat" suits.

Oh! I forgot to mention that, didn't I? Everyone was wearing strange (at least to me) white suits that had a hose going up the back and into their head, completely covered. Through a plastic window, a face would say to me, "Mr. Goodman, do you know why you are here?" I would think, *Hell no, and I would rather be at home.* I can't remember anyone telling me that I was suffering from a very deadly infection. Maybe that happened and I just can't remember, or maybe I didn't understand the severity of the situation. Like I said: Those 30 days at LGH are just a little more than a blur.

In fact, it wasn't until I'd been home for some time that my memory started functioning properly again. I felt good enough to ride my scooter over to Dosie Dough, our local "intelligentsia" coffee shop. One day, I was sitting there at a sidewalk table (they are *all* sidewalk tables these days), sipping on a double espresso with a splash of hot water. Suddenly, I started remembering bits and pieces of my time at LGH. Most prominent among these memories were those from the time I was brought out of my medically induced coma.

One particular recollection is itself a reflection of the unreliability of my memory. It involves one certain doctor, a pulmonary specialist, who looked after me every morning, always coming in really early. He had me on a system that is sometimes called "Hi-Ox." (It had nothing to do with some beast blasted out of its mind on pot.) It was a pressurized oxygen tube that was inserted into the nostrils, and every time I would inhale, this thing would shoot oxygen into my lungs. The problem was, he had to sort of fabricate his own device to insert into my nose. Every morning he would use tape to build up the tubing and then fit it onto my face. There was always a lot of grumbling as he tried to get this thing to work. But while all of this was going on, we had an opportunity to talk.

This man had been in the Air Force and stationed at a base in Colorado. He had a Mustang coupe that he used for going into town. When he received new orders, he found himself shipping out without having made any kind of plans for disposing of this Ford Mustang. I was struggling to stay in the conversation. I was literally fumbling with information about myself. I was trying to remember details about my own car but couldn't get a clear picture in my mind as to what kind of car it was. I drive a nice, cherry, 2006 Mustang GT convertible. It is really a sweet ride and not something that an old hot-rodder like me would forget, but I did.

This same thing happened when I tried to make small talk with the nurses who attended me in their "Moon Suits," as I called them, with the plastic window and face behind it that talked to me. It was as if I had to *explain myself* or somehow, *verify my being*, if you understand what I'm trying to say. I told you about not knowing my own name; well, that same situation carried itself over into the few weeks of recovery immediately after being in the ICU. I had to re-establish my own life! If you have read my book *a. PUZZLED EXISTENCE*, you will discover a full life, numerous college degrees, plenty of world travel, Vietnam combat experiences, etc., etc., *ad nauseam*. Let me tell you that I really had to dig to find the memories, the information about my own existence on this planet Earth. A life of seventy years erased by COVID-19!

My poor, lovely wife was called twice and

told to be ready at a moment's notice to come to the hospital to suit up and to say goodbye to her husband of 34 years. Of course, she was devastated. Anyone would be, under these circumstances. Death via virus from China, where they eat bats and pangolins. Who in their right mind would eat one of those really weird-looking animals? This armor-plated dude runs around the jungle eating bugs. They are strange just to look at, let alone eat. *Tolerance, Jason. Some people have unusual dining habits that involve rare species of animals, some of which are being eaten into extinction. Chomping away on gonads from a hairy thing with four legs and then, bam! The poor thing no longer exists. People do this just to put lead into a penis that has seen its last day a long time ago.* Anyway, enough of the ranting. You aren't reading this book to hear a COVID-19 survivor railing about another country's culinary habits.

I can't go any further with this account of my hospital stay at LGH without sharing my wife's perspective on her experience with the COVID-19 virus. We both wrote articles for the newspaper. Mine was from the viewpoint of a patient, and hers dealt with the other side of this fatal coin toss. Our local newspaper decided to do a story on Teresa and me. One of their star reporters came to our house to photograph and interview us. But the article has yet to appear in print. What started all of this was the way our president (Did you notice I didn't capitalize that word?) ... was talking nonsense about not wearing a mask and saying that this "China Plague," as he was fond of calling it, was a hoax — that is, until *he* got infected.

That is the reason I sat down, wrote my story, and encouraged Teresa to do the same. We wanted people to know that there wasn't any hoax about this stuff — it's very real, and the death toll is still mounting; every single day, a lot of people are dying alone. That was the motivating factor behind my decision to tell you about my experience with this virus. And, the really scary stuff hasn't even been addressed. It's still coming, and it is frightening.

Here is my wife's perspective on dealing with the coronavirus. My inability to remember anything from those first few weeks makes her wrenching experience during those "Lost Thirty Days" even more moving and poignant. So, here it is.

"My husband and I were exposed to COVID-19 on May 13, 2020, by a friend who was unaware he was positive. Within five days, the symptoms began. First was extreme fatigue, followed by headache, fever, and confusion. On the sixth day, Jason was worse. His doctor ordered a test. For the following few days, he rested or slept. We waited for test results. I kept thinking, *If he tests positive, should I drive him to the hospital or call an ambulance?* He was having more difficulty breathing. On Memorial Day morning, his face was ashen, and he was confused. I helped him dress and took him to the VA emergency room. I was not allowed in because of their quarantine protocols. Jason was helped into a wheelchair, and I waited in the car.

"Finally, I was called in — to give my permission to put him on a ventilator. He had deteriorated that fast. I was told that he had COVID-19 and that I probably did, as well. He was admitted, and I drove home, alone. I think I was in shock. I felt numb and overwhelmed. I called my sister, who lives a few miles away, but I isolated myself. I sat home in silence — no TV or radio. I looked at my surroundings and thought, *these things mean nothing to me — without my husband.*

"That afternoon Jason was transferred to another hospital. The ER doctors wanted him to be put on an ECMO machine, which the VA did not have. I heard nothing until the next day, when a doctor called me. He recommended that I get tested for COVID-19. Jason was in critical condition. He was being given convalescent plasma. He was not eligible for the ECMO, because he was older than 65. He was too far into the virus for 'remdesivir.' I was asked about my preferences for life-sustaining measures. The doctor said that I should consider his quality of life if it was necessary for him to go into a nursing home. *He may not make it.* I couldn't see him. He was in isolation. He had gone through a "cytokine storm." He was prone for eight hours and then turned onto his back for eight hours — all the while still on the ventilator. The doctor wanted to do a tracheotomy and get him off the ventilator. The hospital would call me, if necessary, to come in, suit up, and say goodbye to him.

"My days were spent alone. I wasn't hungry. I could not concentrate enough to read. I tested positive for the virus. It left me tired, and now I was depressed. I could hardly wait for nightfall. I wanted it to be dark; perhaps I would sleep. I carried a phone with me, in fear, hoping it would not ring. I thought about funeral arrangements: *Should I have him cremated? What would he want me to do with his ashes? Would I be a burden to my family? Would I stay in this big house?* I felt this weight on my chest. Would Jason die alone?

"Twenty-six days later, my husband was discharged — he had made it through this terrible virus. He'd lost 30 pounds, was weak and pale, but he came home. He would need months of therapy. I am fortunate to have him with me. Yet, I am still afraid. *How close death came to us.* One cannot prepare oneself for the loss of a loved one. The emotions I experienced were feeling overwhelmed, depressed, afraid, and helpless. This virus affects so many people. I think of all the heavy hearts around the world. *All those people dying alone, without their loved ones at their side.* Only someone not touched by the coronavirus could possibly think this is not real. This is real — *very* real. I thank God we made it through."

— Teresa Fee Goodman

It was a time of extreme duress. Teresa spent a good deal of time in our apartment. Her sister, whom she is close to, would not visit for fear of contagion. I can't really blame her, considering the risk. Teresa had this virus, but as is the case with any number of people exposed, her symptoms were milder — nowhere near what happened to me, due to my underlying, pre-existing conditions.

That's something I didn't mention — the pre-existing conditions. In Vietnam, I served on the Mekong River in the Riverine Forces. This exposed us to Agent Orange because they were always spraying the riverbanks to give us a clear line of fire. As a result of that exposure, I have been left with three of the fourteen presumptive conditions associated with this chemical. One of these has to do with lung problems, or COPD, as it is commonly referred to. Naturally, more years than I care to admit of smoking Camel cigarettes didn't help the matter, either. My COPD really came into play with the COVID-19 virus. It is the major reason I ended up in a coma and on a ventilator for 16 days.

One of the main reasons the VA medical center sent me to an outside medical facility was to have them place me on the "ECMO" machine. What "ECMO" stands for is well beyond my pay grade, but I will give you a layman's definition of what this thing does. Basically, it takes your blood out, oxygenates it, and then puts it back into your body — similar to what a dialysis machine would do for a bad set of kidneys. They sent me down there with that intention, but you have to be younger than 65 years for them to consider this application. At the time, I was 70 years old. Maybe the VA just needed to get rid of me because I was severely infected. I don't know, and it doesn't really matter now, anyway.

This is fairly incredible stuff to me as I sit here rehashing the events. I honestly don't know how I survived. I will tell you this: Our spare bedroom is chock full of prayers from well-wishers. I have been saving these because

I don't know how to dispose of them. It might be something like getting rid of used lithium batteries.

In the wake of my near-death struggle with COVID-19, I have experienced a resurgence of my on-again, off-again flirtation with matters of an existential and metaphysical nature. The simple truth of the matter is that I have been an agnostic since I returned from Vietnam. I'm not saying that I am a nihilist, because that is a philosophy that is untenable, according to metaphysical debate. The true definition of a nihilist is someone who doesn't believe in anything, but just the fact that they believe in being a nihilist negates their argument. Philosophy was not one of my majors from my college and university days, but I have read enough to understand the basics and be able to converse with a modicum of intelligence.

As I have mentioned on more than one occasion during this diatribe, I really have only a scant recollection of most of my hospital stay — really just the last few days, when the nurses set up a "video call" with my wife. Other than that, there isn't much to talk about. But the hard fact of the matter is that I was very close to death during that first week and a half.

If that is the case, what would have happened if I had actually died? Where would I have gone? Trust me, I know a little more

The Chronicles of Pain

than most about death.

When I was a young man, I dug graves in a number of cemeteries, so *that* part, I fully understood early in life. Then, in Vietnam, I was responsible for terminating a number of good, honest individuals through what some would call the rigors of war. Though I cannot say that I'm proud of any of that, *it was my job*, as an old Chief Boatswain's Mate explained to me prior to leaving Saigon one day.

And finally, during a summer vacation from writing curriculum while under contract with the Melbourne School system in Australia, I was employed as a funeral parlor worker for Tobin Brothers, one of the largest in that Australian city. My co-worker and I did everything you could imagine that has to do with death except actually making these poor bastards dead. We dressed the dead, transported them, carried them down the aisle, and escorted our late clients to their final rest, either in a crematorium or a dirt burial, if I may borrow an insider's term.

And then there are all of the *personal* near-death experiences I have had over the years. These started with a visit by three doctors to my hospital room on Christmas Day, 1986. They stopped by to inform me that I had less than 10 days to live as a result of my drinking copious amounts of vodka for too many years. This was another little habit that I acquired after my return from Vietnam. A few others add some bulk to the reason why I was hit so hard with COVID-19. One of them was my struggle to stave off the darkness of death from viral pneumonia on more than one occasion.

So, you could say that I have pretty much explored the intricacies of the subject of death — from pretty much every perspective there is. But the question still begs to be answered: What really happened to me in that ICU in May and June of 2020? Even with 10 times the familiarity with death over the average man-on-the-street, I am left with no more insight now into that subject than when I went down the hole of that medically induced coma: My memory of that time period is simply a large blank! If anything, my *wife* died a thousand deaths during this experience — not I. *She* should receive the Nobel Prize for patience and perseverance. *Love During the Time of COVID!!!*

Since I've already related most of what I can remember, I'm going to move into the recuperation stages from coronavirus infection.

I'll never forget the day I got home and finally looked in the mirror. It was downright shocking. My facial skin was all drawn, and I had this full beard. Over the course of those 30 days, I had lost 30 pounds. The face staring back at me from the mirror spoke volumes about disease and subsequent recovery. My fingernails had grown about half an inch. I looked and felt like one of those "Bog People" that had been sacrificed in Ireland. I looked like the crew members from the Franklin expedition lost in the Arctic. It was like looking at a *National Geographic Magazine* cover. From when I got out of ICU and eventually made it home, I'd never seen myself. No one had ever offered me a mirror, and I doubt that I had asked for one, either. In shaving off this hair growth on my face, I blocked the bathroom sink drain, and Teresa had to go buy a small plunger to fix the problem.

I required *two full days* to bring myself into some kind of semblance of who I was before I contracted this virus. It was all quite traumatic. You could almost say that I suffered PTSD again relating to this hospital stay and experienced another near-death chapter in my life. And just think — it's far from over. I had a good belly laugh when Trump announced that he was "cured" of COVID-19. Personally, I am starting to wonder if you *ever* recover from this. And I'll explain why.

There are two flights of steps at my house. We live on the second floor and rent out the downstairs apartment. I had these steps installed, and they have a landing about halfway up, with handrails on both sides all the way up to our apartment. It was set up for my disability because I have issues with my legs and feet. It's from Agent Orange exposure and is called *Early Onset Peripheral Neuropathy* — a gift from Dow Chemical and my time in Vietnam.

As I scaled the first seven steps, it wasn't too bad, but the second seven proved to be a different story. By the time I reached the last three, just before the landing that accommodates our back door, I collapsed. I just couldn't do it. I found myself totally exhausted and out of breath. This was part of the COVID-19 experience. For that first week, I never left my home. The oxygen company had given me a long length of plastic tubing, so I was able to pipe pure oxygen everywhere in my apartment. One length went into the living room, where the "O" generator was located, and another, much longer piece went into my bedroom. I had to use "O" during sleep also — it was a 24/7 type of experience.

One of the nasty characteristics of the COVID-19 virus is that it attacks the lungs and sometimes leaves permanent damage in the form of not being able to retain a high percentage of oxygen in the blood. During those early days, whenever I took off the oxygen, my "O" level would drop very quickly into the 50% range, which is not a good thing to happen. Fortunately, I don't seem to have any permanent damage to my lungs, but it is too early to start shouting in the streets about that.

I'd been home for a few days when my doctor at the VA suggested that I enroll in an "accelerated" rehab program located at the Hershey Medical Center in Hershey, Pennsylvania. Yep, you guessed it — the same town that chocolate bars come from — and I was nuts for going there. Allow me to explain.

After those several days at home, Teresa drove me out to the Hershey Rehab facility. They came out with a wheelchair and piled me into it. When we got to the lobby, they told Teresa that she couldn't go any farther. So here we went again — that loss of communication in a physical sense. They rolled me down the corridor and placed me into a room. I stayed in that same room for seven solid days. My rehab protocol said that I was supposed to have an accelerated program of physical therapy. It called for three solid hours of exercise every day. Then, there was the Occupational Therapy ("OT"), which was designed to help me re-learn how to perform very basic tasks — like tying my shoes, taking a shower, getting out of bed — you know, that sort of critical information. (One of the more sympathetic doctors agreed with me that this was basically a money-making enterprise.)

Now, granted, I *had* tested positive for the COVID-19 virus. That was a simple, clinical conclusion, straight from the facility that treated my infection. I should have been turned away until I had a negative test result. A "positive" COVID-19 status was the reasoning for keeping me locked in my room. Everyone came into that room dressed in their "Hazmat" suits to administer therapy. But this proved to be an exercise in futility. The PT person would have me walk around in circles or lie in bed and do leg exercises. One day the OT lady came in and said, "Do you think you can take a shower?" I told her "Yes," because I had been doing that for the last few days. She told me to go and take a shower. I asked her if she was going to watch, and she said "No." So I went in and took a shower at 1:00 in the afternoon. She sat in the room, doing whatever OT people do when their clients are in the shower!

This "stay" was during the July 4th holiday, so my "therapy" lasted for only four days. On Saturday and Sunday, I was stuck in that room for 24 hours a day. A person would come in three times a day with a tray of food. She would place it by the door in order to save time by not having to change into a "moon suit." Twice a day, they would bring in a paper cup filled with drugs. I was supposed to stay in this program for *14 days*. I said, "No — that's not going to happen." It was a farce, as far as I was concerned.

As you read this book, you will come to realize that I know a little about physical therapy — and this wasn't anything like any other I'd ever had. The therapists would come in late and leave right on the dot at the top of the hour, so, I was getting roughly only 40 minutes of *therapy*. Of course, I'm using that word sarcastically here. My doctor told me that this rehab would be equivalent to 30 days of PT — remember, this was their *accelerated* program. The only thing that was *accelerated* was the federal money going into their checking account.

According to the VA, I am 100% disabled. This means that all of my healthcare costs are covered by the VA. About two weeks after I came home from the Hershey Rehab program, they sent me the bill — more than $13,000. I'd received one week of bad PT and hospital food; they threw in the uncomfortable hospital bed at no additional charge.

Well, I ended up writing them a letter, and they responded with the same blah, blah, blah that administrators are skilled at, like passing the blame by "re-educating" the staff. The thought occurred to me that there was nothing wrong with the *staff*. If anything, this *entire program* should have been called into question.

In the end, I guess the moral of the story is this: If you get this virus and come close to dying from it, then, in recovery, if someone asks you if you want to go to an "accelerated rehab" program, make sure they give you something in writing before you commit to anything. I recently learned that the rehab program at Hershey Medical Center is being operated by an outside entity, "The PennHealth Hershey Group." I'm guessing that they must be supplying space and staff in some capacity that I am not at liberty to comment on, due to the fact that I don't know the particulars of their arrangement. It might be another "pain clinic" situation, like the one I mentioned in previous chapters. Whatever the organizational structure, it doesn't have any bearing on culpability — or the lack thereof.

The crux of the matter had to do with my positive test results. On August 24, 2020, I received the results of my last five COVID-19 tests — they were all *negative*. This diagnosis was very important, as, prior to receiving these test results, I felt like I was walking around with a big scarlet letter on my forehead — "P" for "positive" or "P" for "pariah" — take your pick!

Both Teresa and I wrote stories from our differing perspectives of this ordeal. I jotted down some lines relating to my experience,

The Chronicles of Pain

but the primary reason I took it to the level of writing about it in a book was to send a clear and concise message to everyone out there. I felt the need to warn people that this was not a joke or a hoax. People were going to live or die by their decision to abide by or disregard the CDC guidelines for social distancing and wearing a mask. Take, for example, the annual motorcycle event at Sturgis, South Dakota. There were close to 200,000 people at that gathering in the summer of 2020. When they left, they took the virus with them, causing a major outbreak of COVID-19 in most of the midwestern states, turning the gathering into what the CDC calls a "super spreader" event. That strikes me as a very selfish thing to do. It showed no regard for anyone's health, and that's *wrong*. Under only slightly different circumstances, this would be considered manslaughter, or at least death by misadventure. All of this misery and suffering — just so a handful of people could ride their motorcycles together.

Listen: If you want to gamble with your life and run around without a mask, that's your business. But do *not* — I repeat, do *not* — assume that *my* life is inconsequential. No one is obstructing your freedom. A deadly virus is doing that, and, in order to bring this under control, we all must make some sacrifices. Ask me and I'll tell you — I don't like wearing these stupid masks. I don't appreciate the reduction in my quality of life, the inability to travel, to just sit down at a restaurant and have a nice meal. I object to the confines that this virus has imposed upon my normal lifestyle. But, if we don't try to stem the tide of COVID-19 infection, this will go on and on. It could turn into a common, recurring danger throughout the entire world — like the flu but 100 times more deadly. It will become permanent and constant, no matter what you do or say. This virus may never fade from our lives completely.

In a way, I can see an analogy in the COVID-19 pandemic to the US involvement in the Vietnam war, which was the first to be covered almost in its entirety by members of the press. Every night, people were glued to their television sets, watching a full-scale war take place, without any actors that they could name firsthand. The reporters and journalists never came up the Mekong River, where I served, because we "weren't" in Cambodia at the time. That is what President Nixon was telling everyone in the "world" — contrary to the reality I was living and fighting in.

One of the downsides of war is that someone has to die. Every night people were being told what the body count was on both sides of the Vietnam War, and the common citizen didn't take too kindly to that. For some odd reason, they thought that sending troops halfway around the world would scare the opposition so badly that they would just throw away their guns and run off into the jungle. No one bothered to think that *we* were the invading army, coming into their country and shooting up the place. I would think that if that happened here in the United States, we wouldn't just throw away our guns and run off into the woods somewhere!

The main reason that I have gone off on this digressive tirade has to do with the horror of the television watchers of the Vietnam War back in the 1960s, when they heard about how many of us — the fighting men and women involved with the real war — were being killed or wounded. This really upset people who never bothered to ask why it should have been any different. The equation is simple: We kill them, and they kill us. The only differences were that 1), we killed more of them because of our greater ability to do so with our larger military might, and 2) this was the first conflict in which, because of advances in technology such as the handheld camera, the number of American deaths was readily available *every day*. You didn't even have to leave your house to go out and buy a newspaper for that information. During World War Two, information on casualties was outdated by the time it was reported in a newspaper. With the Vietnam War, that kind of information was delivered straight into your living room — and it was complete and up to date to the very hour in which it was being watched.

The outcome was still the same: A body count was rolled across the bottom of the television screen nightly, the same way they are rolling the numbers with this virus, the COVID-19 pandemic. Why aren't we up in arms about those numbers? As I sit here in front of this typewriter, I'm trying to think of a logical reason why we aren't screaming bloody murder over the number of deaths attributed to this virus. As of this writing, the number is now greater than the number of American deaths in World War One, World War Two, and the Vietnam War — *combined*. Where are the indignant reactions? Where are all of the protestors like we had during the Vietnam War?

Back then, everyone was shouting for us to get the hell out of someone's business that didn't involve us. Why isn't there an equivalent finger sign like the "peace sign" used during those heady days of protest? Could we use a big "V," as Winston Churchill did during *The Big One* — World War Two? Instead of it signifying "victory," it would stand for "virus" — as in *victory over the virus*. Right now, we are being beaten silly by this thing. It's really kicking our ass, and, until January 20, 2021, we had a president who wasn't really doing anything about it.

Am I the only one who doesn't understand the logic to all of this? Have I become delusional, a slight side effect of having had the coronavirus and spending 16 days on a ventilator? Maybe I have permanent brain damage that no one has tested me for. And I won't even go into how this virus seems to be disproportionately impacting people of color. I sincerely hope that isn't true — no one should have to be more likely die from this just because they happen to be a color other than white. Maybe I'm just a 70-year-old naïve individual who doesn't understand the politics of color like our leaders do.

In a few minutes, I'm going to move on into another chapter of this book and, hopefully, interject some humor along the way. I won't apologize for my commentary prior to this point in the book, because it bothers me, as a human being. The argument that no one should have to die needlessly could be made of every war we have ever waged, but that isn't the point here. The point is this: Why wasn't more done to contain this virus? Whose shoulders will the blame settle upon when all is said and done? I could ask even myself: Did *I* do enough to protect other people? I know, beyond a shadow of a doubt, that I brought this thing into my home and infected my own wife. Fortunately, she didn't have to pay the price; I picked up the entire tab for both of us. To defeat this virus will require all of us doing our part — not just Democrats or Republicans — but *all* of us.

If we *all* have to wear face masks, then where is the problem? If that and a little distance helps to stem the tide of this disease, then, again, where is the problem? I don't know about you, but I'm getting tired of my own cooking. (If I say the same thing about my wife's cooking, she'll kill me!) For as much as I liked to complain about airlines, I miss them. (Don't breathe a word to American or United that I said that — they may make their service even worse.) But I want to fly again; I want to see the *tops* of clouds — not just the *bottoms*. I want to hear a different language being spoken at the next table in a real restaurant for a change. I don't want to have to cringe every time I pass someone who is coughing at the grocery store. Come to think of it, I miss being able to find *everything* on my list when I do go to that grocery store — not just *some* of the items. I want to be able to buy drinking water all of the time — not just when it feels *en vogue* to do so.

This virus is killing us and affecting the quality of life in every corner of the world. We have to beat this thing because we have much larger concerns — like rooting out hate groups who want to destroy our constitutional republic and re-install a fascist tyrant.

The Chronicles of Pain

Chapter Five
The Dreaded Follow-Up Visit

The Chronicles of Pain

Just because you spent a week or two in the hospital does not mean you are out of the woods. For the most part, you haven't even found the trail yet! After every surgical intervention, there will be a number of follow-up visits. Hopefully, you won't be sent home with a vacuum pump. They are nice to have for chemistry experiments but not very pleasant in your bedroom, running day and night. There are other horrors, like not responding well to the widget they installed, or hearing a metallic sound every time you jump up and down. (As in "Doctor Howard, Dr. Fine, Doctor Howard," also known as the "Three Stooges." There was one episode where the "patient" gets off the table, and you hear all of these instruments bouncing around inside his stomach. Surgery has come a long way from back then, but if you do hear over the intercom, "Dr. Howard, Dr. Fine, Dr. Howard," run out of that hospital as fast as you can.)

I remember one after-surgery visit that had to do with removing staples. A doctor demonstrated one of his staple guns to me one day. It works basically like the "Arrow T-50" you have somewhere in the garage. The most pronounced difference between that model and the doctor's is its cost and the fact that it is made from plastic. This tool was a one-shot deal. After your doctor is done stapling you up, he tosses the piece into the trash can. Naturally, that staple gun probably carries a price tag of about a thousand bucks. Just think: For that kind of money, you could go out and buy an electric staple gun! Well, of course, I'm making up the price of my doctor's trusty sidearm — all I can do is guess what one of those things cost. If you wish, I could go into a long, boring dissertation, involving reams of technical data from medical-staple-gun manufacturers, which would put us both to sleep. Or I could just say that the price is irrelevant and proceed to relate a true story relating to the removal of staples from my back.

Before I begin, allow me to give a word of caution. Under normal circumstances, you have about 10 to 14 days to get those staples removed. What happens is that the skin begins to grow over the staples, making it more painful to remove them. A little secret is to ask for a topical anesthetic to be applied first, before they start yanking these things out of your flesh. But whatever you do, don't procrastinate on this follow-up visit. The longer you put it off, the more painful it is to have the staples removed.

The other day, I went through my files and actually counted the number of surgeries and other major hospital-related issues in my

The Chronicles of Pain

life to date. The number came to 45 — even *I* was set back by that. There were a few I had completely forgotten, and maybe that lapse in memory wasn't an accident. But, for the record, the story I am about to relate involves one of my back surgeries performed at CMC Hospital in Scranton, Pennsylvania.

On the appointed day, I think it was in 1983, I jumped in the car and drove up the interstate to Scranton for my follow-up visit, primarily for the removal of the staples from the incision in my back. About two weeks had passed since I'd had the operation, and that's why I began this story with a word of caution. The nurse took me into a vacant room and had me sit on a bed while she opened her staple-pulling kit; this is real — there actually exists a toolkit for pulling out surgical staples, and they are throwaway items. She started to pluck the things out, and I could hear them dropping into a little stainless-steel bowl. It reminded me of the old Western movies when the good guy is having a bullet pulled out of his arm with just a piece of wood between his teeth for pain control. You hear the "slug" drop into the metal basin by the doctor's side.

Anyway, she was pulling these things out and started to snicker. Then, she tried to stifle a laugh, and that just led to outright guffawing. Now, keep in mind, I had surpassed the 10-

day window for the removal of these staples, and this was before I knew anything about the use of topical anesthetics. So, this procedure *hurt*. Each one she pulled on was just about killing me, and I didn't see a single tree to chomp down on to ward off the pain. Finally, in my best *Goodfellas* impersonation, when Joe Pesci's character says, "Do I amuse you?" I asked the nurse what the hell was so funny, because, from where I was sitting, there was nothing to laugh about.

The nurse stopped laughing long enough to blurt out, "It looks like Doctor Black has stapled your ass closed!" I would *like* to say that I found this extremely funny at the time. In fact, I would *like* to tell you that I busted a gut laughing out loud. But none of that happened. It probably should have, but it didn't. For this particular surgery, the good doctor had found it necessary to install 84 staples in my back in order to close the wound. I counted every single one of those fucking staples as they came out. My nurse continued to giggle throughout the entire process. So, may this be a warning to anyone who has ever been stapled together: Don't wait until the last minute — time is not on your side with this one. Oh! And ask if the nurse who pulls them out if he or she has ever seen the film *Goodfellas*.

Follow-up visits come in all different shapes

The Chronicles of Pain

and sizes. Sometimes they will want you to come back two or three times. This happened to me recently—just last year, in 2020—with laser surgery for a detached retina. I had to go back to see this guy three times over the course of several months, until I was finally cleared for release. If nothing else, it showed the doctor's commitment to the work, and I would like to think that he took pride in the outcome.

One of the strangest visits that I have ever had happened at the Hershey Medical Center. It was in 2013; I was being seen for a potential surgery on my neck, in the C-5, C-6 and C-7 regions. My arms were going numb, and the medical personnel determined that there was a problem with the nerve trunk in that area. Something was impacting the nerves and causing the numbness. Keep in mind that, by this time, I had been in the care of neurosurgeons for many years; a fairly good number of surgeries had preceded this visit.

My wife and I drove out to the medical facility and were ushered into a small room. We both sat there for some time before the surgeon's assistant came in. He explained that the main man would be in momentarily but that there were a few things that we should be aware of. One of these "rules" had to do with not asking direct questions of the surgeon himself. I found this rather queer; more times than I care to remember, I would ask questions about any given planned intervention. Hell, it was *my* body they were going to cut open and dig around in!

The assistant left, and we sat there for another 15 minutes or so, until the door opened, and they both came into the room. The surgeon sat down at a desk and started to look at the radiologist's report. Then he held a few X-rays up to the light, and then the weirdness started. He would tell the assistant something pertaining to the problem, and then the assistant would turn to us and repeat what the other guy had just said. During this entire exchange, the surgeon never looked directly at me or my wife; he kept his back to us during this entire visit. He told the assistant what he was going to do to fix this problem and how he would accomplish this. The assistant turned to us and repeated the same words. It was one of the damnedest visits with a neurosurgeon that I ever had. When I went to ask something, the assistant stopped me and reminded me of the rule: I was not to address the surgeon directly. The visit lasted only about 10 minutes, and the surgeon just got up and walked out. The assistant stayed long enough to give me the instructions for when I was supposed to return there for this surgery.

I didn't just allow this to slide by. I had to do something to find out why this strange

The Chronicles of Pain

behavior was taking place. It just so happened that the director of the entire department was also going to work on my ulnar nerve at the same time. She was a direct, no-nonsense kind of woman, and, so, I asked her about this guy acting like my wife and I didn't exist. Her response was a shrug of her shoulders and the comment, "What can I say? The guy is a brilliant neurosurgeon, but he has some 'quirks.'" I could probably come up with a few stronger words than "quirky" to describe the weirdness level of that visit. But what else is there to say? The matter was basically closed after the director's comment.

I went ahead and had those surgeries at Hershey Medical Center, though I can say this — the entire process was strange. I've already told you about the tables with wheels, the two swinging doors into the operating theater, and all the rest. This one, though, absolutely took the cake. When my wife dropped me off, she was told that I was going to be prepped for surgery and that there wasn't any need for her to stay around. She was basically given the bum's rush right out of the place.

So, they rolled me in and stuck a few IVs into my arms. I was, of course, wearing the backless gown and lying on a hard stainless-steel table with wheels. When they finally rolled me into the area near the operating rooms, I looked around and realized that I was, maybe, the fifth in line. It reminded me of a busy airport like O'Hare, or Heathrow, with the planes lined up waiting for their turn to take off. There we were, all lined up — five patients wearing those stupid, pooftie hats they place on your head, all lying on tables with wheels, waiting in line to take off. Slowly, the people began to disappear into different operating rooms until it was my turn to lift off into the *Wild Blue Sterile*. Trust me — once they start pumping all of those drugs into your arm — for a few moments, you are definitely flying off into some wild place. Do you remember Aldous Huxley's *Brave New World*, the story about the future society where everyone used "Soma" to soften a cruel reality? Well, that is an apt metaphor for the pipeline into your veins.

If I am not mistaken, four (4) surgeries were performed at the same time. Three were in the C-5, C-6 and C-7 vertebrae region; they had to take out some bone to allow room for the nerves going down my arms. Friction between bone and nerve had been the cause of the numbness in my hand, etc. The fourth surgery was the one on my right arm; it was done to give the ulnar nerve more room. The trouble with that pesky little disorder, called "claw hand," is this: If you don't address it in time, your fingers will fold back. They call this "claw hand," and I know beyond a shadow of a doubt that it happens. My sister-in-law was told that her problem was too old and not a viable candidate for surgery. Her fingers are permanently bent back, into her hand, which renders them just about useless for everyday living. The moral of the story? Have the surgery as soon as possible.

Let's get back to Hershey Medical Center. I went through the PAC unit, was brought down from all of the numbing drugs in my system, and then transported up to a hospital room. They called my wife and told her to be outside the front door at exactly 7:00 a.m. sharp — I was to be discharged at that time. (I will relate the rest of the story shortly.) So, I was stuck in a regular hospital room for the evening. They brought me a tray of gruel; I think it was just a sandwich on fluff bread with a fruit cup and the proverbial Jello.

It was about 11:00 p.m. when I realized that I didn't have a urinal, and I had to go. There was one nurse down the corridor — I could see her shoulder. So, I rang the nurse call button, and nothing happened. I rang that thing several times; she did not budge. Then I shouted out, "Hey, if I don't get a urinal, there will be a puddle on the floor next to my bed." Now that I think of it again, I should have just let loose right there — hang 10 over the side of the bed, between the rails. I shouted out a few more times, all to no avail. She must have had headphones on, because the distance between us was not that great. In the end, I finally got out of bed, which wasn't an easy task, considering that the rails were up. To make matters worse, I was still hooked up to a bunch of different things — monitors, IVs, etc.

With great effort, I "manhauled" all of that equipment across the hall and into the bathroom — just to relieve a natural process. Then, I had to drag it all back and get into bed, no easy task under normal hospital conditions. I never did find out what that nurse was doing. The thought just occurred to me: Maybe it wasn't a real person at all; maybe it was a mannequin or blow-up doll! They probably had to cut back on the personnel budget and dressed up mannequins to look like nurses. Maybe they were dressed-up skeletons.

Early the next morning — I mean *really* early — they woke me up and started to pull off all the wires and IVs. I was handed my clothing and told to get dressed; it seemed there was an urgency to everything they did. Then I was loaded into a wheelchair and rolled into the elevator. I arrived at the sliding glass doors at exactly 7:00 a.m. My wife pulled up at the same moment; they helped me into the car, and away we went. I have never been discharged from a hospital with that kind of German precision. This was my experience with precision surgery, followed by a night in the castle with a beef sandwich, and then the boot at exactly 7:00 a.m. *Thank you. Here's your hat. Don't let the door hit you on the way out!*

Once they start digging around in your lower back, all manner of things could happen. You might come out of surgery with the ability to talk to animals or have an area of your body that can accurately predict the weather. "Yes, sir. My elbow hurts — that means it's going to rain tomorrow, sure enough!" Seriously though, there are a lot of nerves in that area that talk to the brain. Hospital personnel want to know that you can operate your lower 40; they want to make sure it all works down there in the nether regions.

I have actually had that happen. I had a shoulder replacement done, and afterward, I couldn't go! The doctor gave orders to let me go home the next day, *provided* I could go on my own — but it wouldn't work. Man, talk about straining! My head and neck must have been scarlet in color due to the intense pushing. Finally, after many attempts, I almost filled the jug with the golden nectar, and, the next day, *Homeward Bound, Wagons, Ho!!!*

Here is a tip for you if you are determined to

endear yourself to the nursing staff — or wish to make a statement due to some perceived lack of proper respect shown toward yourself. They'll come into your room early in the morning and ask, "Mr. Goodman, have your bowels moved today?" This question is always delivered with a little cheerful lilt. One morning, after a really bad night of insomnia and excessive pain, I answered the question in this manner: "I'm afraid not. They couldn't find the right neighborhood!" Well, that answer immediately erased the lilt in her voice, *and* she squealed on me to Dr. Black. The next day he threatened to cut off my morphine supply unless I was more courteous to his nurses.

The Chronicles of Pain

Chapter Six

Give Us This Day Our Daily *Pain*[4]

---

[4]The author, Jason Goodman, does not give himself enough credit here. He is an experienced world traveler, and, so, I wouldn't have been surprised if he had picked up snippets of different languages. What I *didn't* know about him before this book is that he studied *Latin* for four years (!). [So did I — in addition to six other languages. But I was studying for the ministry of The Lutheran Church-Missouri Synod, and most of those languages were *non-elective, required* courses, so that we could read the Bible in its original languages.] And Latin is, of course, the rock-solid foundation for most of the Romance languages of Europe — including French.

In the title of this chapter, there lies a delicious little linguistic irony — and, now, I realize that Jason was fully conscious of it. He took a verse from the Bible — the famous lines that Jesus used to teach his disciples how to pray, which later became known as "The Lord's Prayer" (found in both Matthew 6:9 and in Luke 11:2). Jason took the "Give us this day our daily bread" part and replaced the word "bread" with "pain." Do you know what the French word for "bread" is? *Le pain.* I kid you not. [Frank W. Kresen — editor]

The Chronicles of Pain

Back in the old days, before dirt was invented, I used to be young and stupid. Some would argue that I am merely old and stupid now, but that is still up to the courts to decide, and I can't comment due to ongoing litigation. Another important thing to factor in is my use of alcohol for recreational purposes in those days. The truth is a little more involved. I returned from Vietnam with some unresolved issues that pretty much equated to throwing gasoline on a burning fire when I indulged in the use of alcoholic beverages. Thankfully, all of that is solidly behind me and has been for more than 34 years, but there were some good times. If you are interested, there are two books of short stories that I've written: *Urban Gothic 1* and *Urban Gothic 2*. There are all factually based, which is another way of saying that they actually happened. The material can be a little adult-themed at times, but the stories are *very* funny. So, with that said, I will try to weave in a true story that is somehow related to the subject of this book — *pain*.

Between Vietnam and rheumatoid arthritis, I have had to replace three major bone joints. My right knee was done twice. Then another ortho man debrided my patella, aka, kneecap. The reason I had to have my right knee replaced twice is an interesting story.

The orthopedic department at the Veterans Hospital in Lebanon, Pennsylvania, specializes in joint replacement. I went out there, and they took a few black-and-white X-rays of my right knee. The doctor said, "Your knee joint is no longer round; it has facets, and that may be the source of your pain." They set me up for surgery, and I went in and had it done. The knee is a difficult surgery to recuperate from. It requires an iron will and determination to attend all of the 15 weeks of PT, and that includes any number of exercises they want you to do at home in between sessions. And it all hurts like hell. They say that the only thing worse than a knee replacement is having your shoulders replaced.

Well, guess what? I have had both of those done, also.

But back to the knee joint. I did everything that was asked of me, and the pain subsided and then went away — at least the worst of it. It was 2010 by the time I was released from PT and received my walking papers, my wife and I went down to Mexico. We used to spend the winters there. One day, I was on a Mexican bus when it hit the deepest pothole that I have ever seen. My leg, the one with the brand-new knee, had to absorb all of the shock. It went from my right foot up and out the top of my head. As soon as I stepped out onto the sidewalk, I knew something was busted in my right knee. So, I went and bought a cheap cane and managed to stay the rest of our pre-paid weeks in Puerto Vallarta.

As soon as I got back, I went out to the VAMC at Lebanon and asked what had happened. They did X-rays, gamma rays, and Corvette Stingrays, and then told me, "We have to go in there again!!!" And in they went. It was another four-hour surgery, and I ended up in the same machine that automatically flexes your knee 24/7 while you lie in bed. This isn't really pleasant because it hurts like hell.

The next day, my orthopedic surgeon walked into my room and proceeded to explain to me what happened. He said that there is this plastic plate that fits over the tibia; the titanium knee joint "rides" on this plate. He then started to think out loud. His next comment was, "That plate fit so well in there. I mean, it was really tight. I decided not to use medical adhesive on it to hold it in place. I don't understand what could have happened…"

As I was lying in that bed, with this humming and clicking device flexing my knee, which hurt with every completed circuit, I was rolling over in my head this doctor's comment about not using medical adhesive. I kept asking why he hadn't used glue on this knee replacement. Finally, I worked up enough courage to ask him. "Doctor, do you mean to tell me that I'm here, going through another complete knee replacement because you decided not to glue the thing together?"

He basically told me *yes* and repeated the part about how well the plate fit without the adhesive. Then he went on to say something about the buses in Mexico, more or less implying that *I* was the reason this knee joint failed. His logic was quite simple: American tourists don't ride the bus in Mexico; they *always* use cabs!

I recovered from that surgery but still had some significant pain issues. It had gotten so bad that I had to walk with a cane. Every time I went to see my "ortho-man-without-adhesive," he would tell me it was in my head. To make a long, four-year story short, this guy retired (and had to have a knee replaced), and another big dog was on the porch, a young guy with an Italian name. I went to see him; he stuck the X-ray up on the lighted board, rubbed his chin, pointed, and said, "There is your problem — right there. Your patella needs to be debrided."

I asked what that entailed. He told me that they would cut the knee open, pull out the patella and flip it over, scrape off the bony buildup, glue on a nice, smooth piece of plastic, flip the kneecap back over, and stitch it all up. He told me that the last thing they wanted was

The Chronicles of Pain

to damage the tendons — the original kneecap works the best. The day after this surgery, he said, "Oh, by the way, you'll never guess what I dug out of your knee: a piece of shrapnel. It was small, but it was in there all of those years, 50 to be exact!"

You may be wondering about some of my stories, and I assure you that you aren't alone. I often wonder about them myself. Seriously, though, my painful mistakes are yours to avoid for the price of this book. Those four years of pain and use of a cane weren't in my head. I know my own body, and I knew that something was wrong with it. No doctor can flat out dismiss your concern by saying it's in your own head. I was dealing with the Veterans Administration healthcare program for veterans, who operate on an entirely different schedule than the people outside that system. I *had* to deal with the "glueless ortho-man"; my choices were quite limited at that time.

But *yours* don't have to be. Even the VA has changed their policies, allowing one to go outside the system. My knee was replaced in early 2009. Fortunately, I won't have to go through the "in your head" diagnoses. I have come to understand one thing clearly: Doctors are *not* gods!

It was 1983. I had just gone through my second divorce and basically lost everything in the process. I ended up with a crapped-out pickup truck and a one-room cabin on the beach in a little South Florida neighborhood that was called. "Briney Breezes." It sounds rather idyllic, doesn't it? Well, if the situation had been closer to normal, it would have been. There were four of these little cabins; they all had tiny kitchens and bathrooms and one great room. We're talking about less than 200 square feet in total.

I was working for an excavating company out of Fort Lauderdale, operating heavy equipment, mostly very large bulldozers. I had worked for my immediate boss before, with a different outfit. He was up to his neck in a job that was way behind schedule, and I helped him out of a fix, you might say, by basically doing my job. Allow me to add at this point that this guy was a born-again Christian, which didn't affect me one way or the other. A man's beliefs are his own, as far as I am concerned, though this *is* pertinent to the story.

One night, my ex-girlfriend, the person who'd helped expedite my trip to divorce court, brought a friend of hers and a big bottle of cheap vodka to my beach cabin. Did I tell you that these four cabins were situated in a grove of Australian pine trees about 100 yards from the beach? I mention that because I would get visitors simply because it was hard to park

The Chronicles of Pain

near this particular beach. But that night, it was a different type of visit. The "friend" she had tagging along was an enforcer for some gang up north. What little I gleaned was that he had to leave town in a hurry for whatever enforcers do in their spare time.

The party of three started out quite amiable enough, with drinks and small talk, but that quickly changed in direct proportion to the amount of vodka that was consumed, and a fight broke out. He and I went rolling around in this tiny little house, busting up the place, punching each other whenever an arm was clear of a closet or kitchen. We broke even on injuries — he left with a busted eye, and I had three broken ribs.

The next day, I showed up for work, as usual, but I have to admit that I wasn't really up to the task of wrestling this big Caterpillar bulldozer around all day. So, I called in to the office and told them that I'd fallen down some stairs and busted a few ribs the night before. My boss told me to stay there until he arrived. It was sheer agony trying to push a pile of sand up a hill with this huge machine until he eventually showed up. It started to rain, and he invited me to sit in his car. I will never forget the image of the windshield wipers swooshing back and forth while we spoke. He explained to me that this job was way behind schedule and that it was costing the company a zillion dollars a day because of that and would I please stay there and push sand up that hill. I kept trying to tell him that it was painful to breathe and that I was in some serious pain.

With that, he actually did the following: The guy "laid hands" on me and started to pray to God to fix my ribs so that I could continue pushing that sand around all day because he, my boss, was in a jam because he'd let the job get behind schedule. Then — I kid you not — he started to *talk in tongues*. There I sat, watching the windshield wipers go back and forth while this guy had his hands on me, talking in tongues, trying to heal my three broken ribs so that I could manhandle this bulldozer for the rest of the day, *in the rain*, no less.

After he came out of his little trance, he told me to go forth and bulldoze. He was confident that, within 30 minutes, my ribs would be healed, and I would happily stay the rest of the day, shoving sand up a hill with a Caterpillar bulldozer. I watched him drive away and then tried several times to climb back up onto this lump of pig iron with a soul. Well, guess what happened? I stayed for about an hour and then turned the machine off, got into my old, crapped-out pickup truck and drove home — only to find out that I was being evicted.

The speaking in tongues and laying on of

hands had not reduced my pain in the least. I have no desire to start a debate about the efficacy of prayer, nor am I tossing any barbs at anyone's belief system. All I am trying to say is this: Prayer does not necessarily relieve pain. That is the outcome of my experiences with the subject, and there are a few others that I will not go into at this time. The way I see it, one story about that form of pain relief is enough for one day, or at least one chapter.

Own your pain. Do you remember this from my Charleston Pain Clinic experience? Well, it's true — I must *own my pain* every day. In about an hour or so, I will be at a pulmonary-rehabilitation clinic, doing very strenuous exercises. This therapist is a man-killer; she will have me going like crazy on an elliptical machine, while she checks my oxygen percentages and my heart rate. This exercise will kill me with pain; when I finish, I will barely be able to walk to the elevator, but I won't show her that. I'm there voluntarily for treatment of post-COVID-19 lung dysfunction. This treatment is actually improving my lung capacity, and I'm seeing and feeling actual improvement. Why would I want to allow my old, constant, chronic pain stand in the way of that? I won't — because they are two entirely different things.

Another benefit is that I have a gym at

my disposal. Just recently, our governor here in Pennsylvania closed all of the gyms due to the virus uptick, but I have one at my disposal three times a week. This is a win-win situation for both my chronic pain and my COVID-19 recovery. You are undoubtedly trying to figure out why I'm excited about using a gym for chronic pain. The answer is simple: I have to!

There are numerous books and papers on the subject of exercise and its benefits. I can only comment on how it has affected me over the years. I began in the mid-1980s with trainers and the gym culture. My doctors at the time knew that I would benefit from a planned exercise regimen, and I did. The increased strength I achieved helped me to deal with the chronic pain — not to mention what it did for my outlook. Over a period of time, I realized that I could actually reduce my dependence on opioid medications to a certain degree. It usually worked like this: During the day, I felt fairly good. I could deal with the chronic pain pretty well, but, in the evening, the invoice came due, and I needed that extra boost to get through the evening hours.

Today, I can go into a gym and establish a schedule of exercise for myself. This is possible only because of the many years I spent working with good trainers who would show me what to do; they always had a plan. I would not suggest just popping into a gym somewhere wearing a nice, new, tight-fitting spandex outfit and start throwing pig iron around. You will probably do more damage than good to your body and increase your pain load. You will need a structured program initially, with a good trainer who is familiar with chronic-pain individuals and their needs. You can find these people in most well-run gyms, but it is imperative that you find the *right* trainer, as suggested.

You must start slowly and work up to a more strenuous routine. This could take three to four weeks; during that early period, you will experience more pain in areas of your body where there wasn't any before. That's par for the course; you will be awakening muscles that have been there all along but that have not been asked to do anything substantial. This is the key to a good program — building up those muscles that haven't been used before. It will definitely help you in the long run. For example, most of my pain derives from the back surgeries I have endured. By working the back muscles around those weakened spots, the load will be spread out a bit. Those newly introduced muscles will carry more of the load and, in turn, help relieve some of the pain.

At this stage, I would not suggest running home and throwing out all of your pain meds. You will still need to rely upon these, but maybe to a lesser extent. The secret is to *stay with it*. When you wake up in the morning and your brain is telling you to skip this session, that is the most important time to go to the gym. Establish a three-days-a-week routine, and stay with it, because it will produce *other* beneficial results — mainly in your attitude. You cannot allow yourself to succumb to your pain. If you do that, a number of ominous behaviors will set in, the first being complaints. You will start complaining more and flying off the handle at everyone around you. Your constant complaints will not endear you to anyone within earshot — you will simply devolve into a royal pain in the ass. I used the term "royal" because my wife is making us watch another season of *The Crown*. God! Talk about a royal pain in the ass! Just take in that series if you need further definition of the term. Actually, it *is* a good series to watch.

As I mentioned a number of times, you must *own your pain*. It is yours, and no one can take it from you or help relieve the daily burden. I have already spoken about suicidal ideation that proceeds from lost hope — the hope that this will be lifted and that your life will return to normal. What exactly is *normal*? Does anyone really know? I doubt it, because what is normal for one person does not always translate into another's daily life. We all carry some kind of

The Chronicles of Pain

pain, be it mental, physical, or even emotional. Each set of circumstances translates into an individual response; that response can be in the form of agony, distress, or, in my case, mind-numbing physical pain.

Fortunately, I have a wife who loves me. Don't ask me to explain her motives, but the fact of the matter is that she does. That helps me in the emotional sense, because I can rely on her affection, no matter what. But, if I were to bring home the burden of chronic pain every day and lay it at her feet, I would render her impotent. She can't fix it or even relate to what it really means to live with chronic pain. It is not her business to understand that condition if she isn't personally involved in the daily life of pain. What would I gain by making her existence miserable due to my refusal to deal with the problem? *Own your pain!*

Believe me, your face will tell someone who loves you everything they need to know about your pain level. Allow that knowledge to be mostly a *silent* understanding. Meet the obvious question with a simplistic response, such as, "Yes, dear. It's a bad day." Then let it go at that. People will respect you more when you own your pain. They know you are hurting, but what can they do about it? Nothing. So, answer that question *for* them: "Yes, it's been a bad day. Now, what's for dinner?"

I returned from Vietnam in 1970. For the next 30 years, I never dealt with the unresolved issues that I experienced in combat during that war. During those years, it was not the easiest thing to talk about. No one wanted to hear about Vietnam — not even other people who'd served in that conflict. There seemed to be this prevailing feeling that we, collectively, had "lost" that war. The people at home didn't want to be reminded of their own guilt, and they sure as hell didn't want you, the returned serviceman, reminding them of that guilt! So, I suffered in silence, but the difference was this: I did not *own* my experiences! They were attached to something that I did not understand. It was an unresolved issue that could not be dealt with internally. I needed outside help; I needed someone else to explain the anger. I required another person to tell me what it was that I did over there and why it was necessary.

That help did not come until the early '90s, when I sought out clinical psychology. This came in the form of a doctor at the Veterans Hospital in Wilkes-Barre, Pennsylvania. He was an old Jewish psychologist who specialized in working with combat veterans. I saw this person on and off for a period of 10 years, and he helped me resolve these issues and move on with my life.

You are undoubtedly asking yourself why I

even bring up this topic in a book about chronic pain. During those 30 years prior to seeking out the help I needed, I was married twice. You could say that I didn't *marry* those women as much as I *took them hostage*. I was not the man that I am today, because, back then, I never said a word about Vietnam to anyone. So, during those ill-fated marriages, I made those individuals miserable with my mood swings and fits of anger.

Do you see the correlation that I'm getting at here? I didn't *own my issues* from Vietnam, because I was the only one trying to resolve them. I did not have the benefit of someone explaining to me in simple terms how to understand what it was that I was feeling. Owning that entire experience, through the help of an outside observer, was finally achieved 30 years after the fact. But, in the meantime, I made a lot of people — people who actually *cared* for me — impotent and miserable because they didn't understand what it was that made me act the way I did toward them. Today, when someone says, "Thank you for your service," I understand how to respond, because I own my entire experience with regard to that war. Respect is offered, and respect is given in return. I'm capable of doing that because I accepted and educated myself about those issues.

This same thing applies to my chronic pain — I understand it, I live with it, and I respect the feelings of those around me regarding how to deal with it. I am the *sole owner* of this condition referred to as chronic physical pain.

When you arrive at this destination — being the sole owner of chronic pain — your options are limited. You can either accept the fact and live with it, using everything at your disposal to deal with this on a daily basis, or you can take the way-more-extreme measure of taking your own life with the express intent of being without pain. These are the options available to people like us. One requires understanding of the situation; the other simply says, "No, I'm not going to deal with this any longer!" When you employ *that* solution, you must take into consideration a myriad of complications. Depending upon the methodology used, you are going to leave some kind of mess for someone else to clean up. Whether it be gray matter splashed all over the sofa or a coroner's report that would make a life insurance company happy, the outcome is still the same. *You are without pain, but everyone you have left behind will inherit their own form of the same.* So, careful consideration must go into this decision before it is acted upon, unless you *just don't care*. With *that* response, there is no one who can argue the point.

The Chronicles of Pain

My recommendation would be to explore every avenue prior to acting hastily. We have to educate ourselves to everything that is out there for our benefit. Recently, I have begun looking at the advances in stem-cell research with rebuilding lung tissue. It might hold out some promise for this COPD that I smoked myself into. Someday in the near future, I may be able to have stem cells injected into my chest, and, *Voila!* New lungs.

Maybe the same could be done for my chronic pain. Who knows? In that same future, there could be a procedure that would just remove all of the pain. Of course, these all represent *long-term* solutions, whereas taking myself out is just a *short-term* resolution to an ongoing problem. It is my decision and mine alone. Granted, living in constant pain is not what anyone would consider to be a rosy life, but the operative word here is *living*, as opposed to being deceased. That, my friends, is the *final* resolution. (There was another term I was tempted to use just then, but the Third Reich rendered that to infamy for all time. So, I will stick with the terminology that I have employed here.)

Pain affects everyone differently. Some people can just shrug it off and keep going. Others have to sit down and never get back up again. And then there is the fighting approach.

This is the avenue that I have embarked on. I fight this thing every day, and I am determined not to allow this pain to take over my life. I do whatever is necessary to live fully for another day. In the end, that is all we are ever guaranteed — just *today*, this 24-hour period. I was once told that the difference between projecting and planning is just one word: *Outcome!* When I start to *plan* the outcome of anything, then I'm projecting. Projection is based on something that is supposed to happen in a prescribed way. But when you live in chronic pain, you can't always live in that confidence. Things have a way of inserting themselves into our lives regardless of our plans to the contrary.

The key to living with chronic pain is just that — *living*! I try to squeeze every droplet out of every day, knowing that my pain hasn't taken more — not even a *speck* more — of my life than it is entitled to. *I* get to decide how many rights my pain can have. I do know this: Pain doesn't have any right to the rest of my life. It is *mine*, and I will remain very selfish with every day that fate has in store for me. Chronic pain cannot dominate my life. Only *I* can allow that to happen, and I refuse, on a daily basis, to give this entity anything that belongs to me. I am well aware and have completely accepted the fact that I live in pain. So what? It cannot consume my life unless I give it my permission. That will never happen because I *own my pain*!

The End (for now!)

Index of medical procedures:

The Chronicles of Pain

#:	Procedure:	Date:
5	Back surgeries (lower) Laminectomies — L-1, 2, 3, 4, 5. S1 & S2	1986, 87, 88 1990, 01, 02
1	Vasectomy 1985	
1	Fusion @ L-4 & L-5	1993
2	Install and removal of a subcutaneous morphine delivery system	1996
1	Removal of nerve root tumor 1994	
4	Microlaminectomies — C-4, 5, 6, 7.	2009
3	Ulnar nerve surgeries	1997, 98, 2009
2	Colon polyp removal (Major)	2012, 13
3	Right knee joint replacement Failed knee replacement Right patella de-briding	2008 2008 2012
2	Right and left shoulder joint replacements	2014 2015
2	Abdominal aneurism repair Vascular correction of same.	2012 2019

26 subtotal

#:	**Dental procedures:**	**Date:**
3	Dental implants	1996, 97
3	Dental implants—replacements	2015, 16, 17
6	Bone grafts	1996, 97, 98 2015, 16, 2020
1	Left lower jaw bone replacement	2018
2	Sinus lift procedures	2019, 2021

41 subtotal

#:	**Vision/eye surgery:**	**Date:**
1	Laser stigma correction	2018
1	Cataract removal w/ lens replacement	2018
2	Detached retina repairs	2019, 20

The total number of medical interventions to date: 45.

The Chronicles of Pain

The purpose for listing all of these medical interventions was to drive home the fact that I have been through the mill when it comes to hospitalizations. Every one of the procedures that are listed involved a hospital stay for varying lengths of time. The dental and eye procedures may have required only a one-day visit, but trust me, they were more than just simple things. When they rebuilt my lower jawbone, I spent three hours in that dental chair, under full operating-room protocol. Everyone who participated was fully gowned, and there was a person monitoring my vital signs at all times.

Another aspect to take into account would be the long, protracted periods of physical therapy that would accompany major back or joint-replacement surgery. When I had that fusion of my lower back vertebrae, it entailed the wearing of a "Jewett" brace for several months. I even attended a few group sessions of "Jewett-brace" wearers. These were weekly meetings for individuals who'd had fusion surgery and were forced to wear that medieval contraption. It was designed to keep your spinal column perfectly straight at all times, but it was mind-numbing in its application. This thing could easily replace Hell's fires any day of the week in terms of sheer torture. Ask anyone who has gone through that, and they will undoubtedly tell you the same thing that I have just related. My joint replacements required upwards of 15 weeks of PT, twice a week, and sometimes three times per week.

Everything above just adds exponentially to the pain level of the day. After you get home is when the pain really starts. These are my personal credentials when it comes to chronic pain and any related matters, such as extended hospital stays.

The Chronicles of Pain

ACKNOWLEDGMENTS:

After having more than 40 procedures, my itinerary of hospitals has grown over the years; some warrant great helpings of praise, while others are better left unmentioned. But a hospital is more than a set of buildings with a lot of things on wheels rolling around. Really good hospitals are made up of really outstanding individuals, be they doctors, nurses, administrators, or even the billing department. That last one we will not be going into in any detail, at least not in this edition.

I can't help but notice that there has been a gradual change in the care given at hospitals over the years. I would attribute that to the health-insurance industry more than any other factor. I know for a fact that they limit the number of minutes a doctor can spend with his patient. In some facilities, the professional staff barely have enough time to write up their reports before another patient knocks on their door. I was told recently that they wanted doctors to see a patient every 15 minutes, a Herculean task under normal circumstances — let alone in a patient-provider relationship. I am not sure that the path we are on in relation to these imposed time restraints is a good one. It may be beneficial to the health-insurance company's bottom line but leaves much to be desired when it involves patients being herded through on a production line. I actually made a reference to this type of medical practice during my experience at the Hershey Medical Center. It was like watching them assemble a Mercedes Benz automobile in Germany. (That last reference came from watching a "YouTube" video dealing with the same!)

The unfortunate thing about all of this is the knowledge that it will never return to those "good old days," when doctors actually had the time to make house calls. And, they usually had medications in their bag that they would dispense in something that looked like a small matchbox. There was usually no charge because they were free samples.

Well, I think that it may be necessary to return my trusty soapbox to its little location beneath the steps and get on with the subject of acknowledgments. Before I go any further with the individual accolades, allow me to list some, if not all, of the hospitals that I have been a patient in.

The Chronicles of Pain

Nesbitt Memorial Hospital Kingston, PA	1950 & 52
Oakland Naval Hospital Oakland, CA	1970
Community Medical Center Scranton, PA	1986, 88, 1990 1991, 92, 2003
Boca Raton Regional Hospital Boca Raton, FL	1988
Depoo Hospital Key West, FL	1984, 84
Hospital San Javier Marina Puerto Vallarta, Mexico	2008
Veterans Administration Medical Center Lebanon, PA	2006, current
Veterans Administration Hospital Philadelphia, PA	2011
Veterans Administration Hospital New York, NY	1992, 93
Veterans Administration Hospital Wilkes-Barre, PA	1996 to 2006
Homestead Baptist Hospital Homestead, FL	1983
Roper Hospital Charleston, SC	1990 to 1996

Mayo General Hospital Castlebar, Ireland	2018
Galway Clinic Galway, Ireland	2010
Royal Melbourne Hospital Melbourne, Australia	1976, 77
Lancaster General Hospital Lancaster, PA	2019 & 2020

The Chronicles of Pain

I felt that it wasn't prudent to list all of the clinics that I have been in over the years. In Vietnam, I was seen on a regular basis at the clinics in Saigon and Vung Tau, due to injuries sustained while under hostile fire. In 1970, they were having a tough time replacing experienced people to carry on that war. So, unless your leg went missing, or other parts of your anatomy seemed to disappear, they would usually patch you up and send you back into the fray. Naturally, you always had your little bottle of Darvon capsules when you left; that was pretty much standard *modus operandi* back in those days.

Setting all of that aside, allow me to begin to thank everyone involved in making this book available. You would be surprised how many individuals it takes to create a published literary work, and for that reason, I would be remiss not to extend my sincere thanks to everyone involved.

For reasons of personal security, I cannot allow an acknowledgment page to be printed without my sincere and heartfelt thank-you to my wife and partner in life, Teresa. She has replaced my mother, Mary T., as the driving force in my existence. All of the better qualities that I exhibit are due to the constant input of my wife.

Frank Kresen and his capable wife, Kim,

deserve a special word of gratitude from me because they make this entire book legible. Without them, every other word in this manuscript would be damaged in some way, and there would not be any commas left for anyone else to use. I tend to monopolize every comma that has ever been created.

Throughout my journey into the medical profession, I can assure you that there have been doctors and nurses who have literally saved my life. By saying "saved my life," I mean that in a strict sense of the word. There have been doctors of medicine, of the body and its internal workings, and then there have been the doctors of the mind I have dealt with who talked me out of a few very bad ideas over the years. I have also omitted and must acknowledge the staff of three treatment hospitals that I have been a patient in. You cannot live in chronic pain without addressing the abuse of alcohol and other drugs just to have a moment's relief, something to make your body and mind numb. But all of these things have dire consequences. In 1986 on Christmas morning, I had three doctors with clipboards come into my hospital room to tell me that I may have 10 more days to live, due to the ravages of unchecked alcoholism. They then added insult to injury by telling me that I was not a good subject for organ harvesting, due to the toxicity of my blood. Over the span of these pages, I have touched upon the practice of using alcohol as a treatment for chronic pain. If you're considering this, please reconsider. It is a slippery slope and best left unexplored. Why add an entire new dimension to an already-monumental problem that must be dealt with on a daily basis?

Another of the most important factors in treating chronic pain is heartfelt love. We must have people who care for us and provide that extra impetus to keep going another day. Excessive drinking will drive that love away. Let me just say this, from my own personal experience: That is the last thing you would want to do to survive.

Finally, I would like to thank you, the reader, for acquiring my book. I sincerely hope that my words have helped at least one individual suffering from the same condition that I have: Getting through another day. And maybe, just maybe, I have cracked a smile on a few grim faces in the process.

Jason P. Goodman

The Chronicles of Pain

Made in the USA
Middletown, DE
08 August 2023